IN THE
BONESETTER'S
WAITING-ROOM

AARATHI PRASAD was born in London to an Indian mother and Trinidadian father, and was educated in the West Indies and the UK. After a PhD in genetics she worked in research, policy and communication, presenting documentaries for the BBC, Channel 4, National Geographic and the Discovery Channel. She is the author of *Like a Virgin: How Science is Redesigning the Rules of Sex* and works at University College London.

IN THE BONESETTER'S WAITING-ROOM

TRAVELS THROUGH INDIAN MEDICINE

AARATHI PRASAD

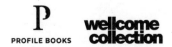

PROFILE BOOKS

wellcome collection

This paperback edition published in 2017

First published in Great Britain in 2016 by
PROFILE BOOKS LTD
3 Holford Yard
Bevin Way
London
WC1X 9HD
www.profilebooks.com

Published in association with Wellcome Collection

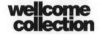

183 Euston Road
London NW1 2BE
www.wellcomecollection.org

Wellcome Collection is the free museum and library for
the incurably curious. It explores the connections between
medicine, life and art in the past, present and future. It is part
of Wellcome, a global charitable foundation that exists to
improve health for everyone by helping great ideas to thrive.

A CIP catalogue record for this book is available from the
British Library.

ISBN 978 1 78125 487 5
eISBN 978 1 78283 178 5

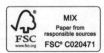

For Tara, my star.

Contents

	Introduction	I
I	Depressed in Dharavi	12
2	Bollywood Bodies	40
3	Knowledge for Long Life	63
4	The Heart of the Matter	94
5	Blood, Bile, Bone	112
6	The Fish Doctors	136
7	The Mother Goddess	160
8	Rewiring the Brain	187
	Acknowledgements	211

The real voyage of discovery consists not in seeking new landscapes, but in having new eyes.

MARCEL PROUST

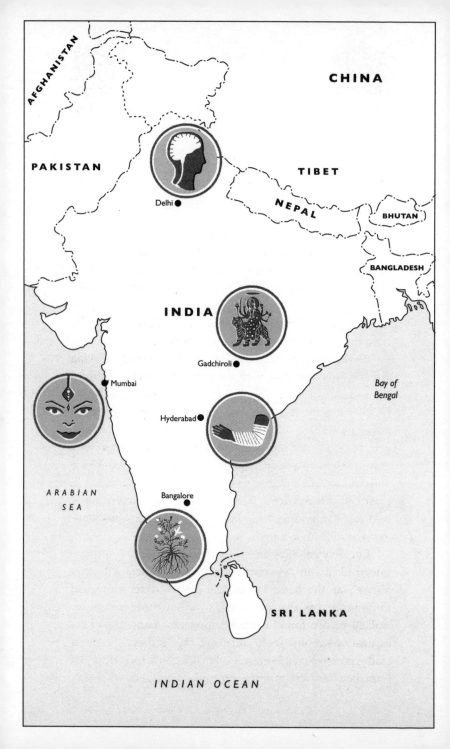

Introduction

EARLY ONE SUNDAY MORNING, I got into a taxi headed for
Bangalore's City Market. A friend of mine, an artist who
had created a montage of Indian medicinal plants for London's Natural History Museum, told me to meet him there.
'They sell everything,' Sunoj said, 'even things you wonder
how anyone could ever need.' I was intrigued.

By the time I got there the streets were already heaving
with crowds bartering with vendors while trying to avoid
the constant flow of people, rickshaws, cows grazing on
rubbish and the threat of rain. Sunoj was right about the
offerings – there were stripped wires and light switches;
decades-old badminton shuttlecocks made of real cork and
goose feathers; antique brass ornaments and paintings;
ancient coins of dubious provenance, Bakelite telephones,
plastic shoes and semi-precious gems. Sometimes, Sunoj
told me, if you looked carefully, there were the most wonderful curios to be found.

But we were browsing with a purpose: here, Sunoj had
informed me, in the centre of the subcontinent's 'Silicon
Valley', at the heart of India's home of technological
innovation, was also an ancient world of medicine. As we
walked on we found a man selling talismans to protect
against scorpions, snake bite and the 'evil-eye'; another
stall – probably the busiest – offered a black rock from the
Himalayas, which, mixed with milk, would cure digestive

difficulties and back pain. There was a young woman with bottles of dried Ayurvedic herbs to be mixed with coconut oil, who released her Rapunzel-like locks as I talked to her, to prove the power of her herbal hair oil. 'Look,' she said, 'look how long it has grown in a year.' I asked her how long it was to start with. She indicated a very short bob, around the level of her ears. 'I cut my hair to sell it,' she continued, 'and with this oil, look how fast and beautifully it grows!' I was sure there'd be a stall selling human hair around the next corner, though not hers; not just yet.

I took her leaflet and walked to another area of the market where a man had pitched a large parasol, an old barber's chair and a cabinet covered with surgical tools, a box full of teeth and several sets of dentures. Sunoj was impressed. 'Much better equipped than he was last time I came,' he told me. 'But even then he had plenty of customers.'

When I got home, I told my mother about the street dentist. 'Did he have his monkey with him?' she asked, as if it were the most natural thing in the world. 'Why on earth would he have a monkey?' I asked. 'Because they have a very strong grip. When I was a child, street dentists used to have monkeys to help them.'

My mother was born in Bangalore in 1947, a few months before India became independent. In Delhi, even as thousands of refugees created by the subcontinent's partition into India and East and West Pakistan were still housed in makeshift camps around the city, long-discussed blueprints for the nation's new policies were being moulded. Among the goals were sustained economic development, education for the masses and healthcare for all. To many Indians, this meant making use not only of Western drugs and procedures but also of the many and varied traditional systems that had been practised across the country for centuries.

Charged with assisting the transition of India and Pakistan to independence, the interim government convened its first health ministers' conference. As a result, my mother's father, a doctor of Ayurvedic medicine, was appointed secretary to the Chopra Committee, set up to make recommendations on both training and the synthesis of Indian (principally Ayurveda and the Greco-Arabic Unani) and Western medicine. Yet, despite the committee's best efforts, it would be around another fifty years before the government of India would create a department for traditional medicines under its Ministry of Health.

Today, medicine in India continues to be a multidisciplinary system in which there are not just three, as my grandpa and his colleagues were juggling, but seven officially recognised types of healthcare. The one with which Westerners are most familiar is variously called English, allopathic, Western, modern or biomedicine. Their doctors are referred to as MBBS doctors, after the name of the internationally accepted university qualification (Bachelor of Medicine, Bachelor of Surgery) for medical students.

Three others – Ayurveda, Yoga and Siddha – are Indian by birth. Unani, also of ancient origin, is Greek (via the Arab world) and the two most recent – Homoeopathy and Naturopathy – originated in nineteenth-century Europe. The collective term for this sextet of traditional systems is AYUSH, derived from the Sanskrit for 'long life' but is also an acronym of (most of) their initials.

Though allopathic medicine and AYUSH are based on vastly different principles, in practice doctors often have recourse to both systems. There are close to 400 MBBS medical schools in India, a mixture of highly competitive state colleges and expensive private ones, which prepare Indian doctors for mainstream medical careers in India. Alongside these mainstream schools are 500 universities and specialist medical colleges producing AYUSH graduates who are also taught relevant biomedical subjects – anatomy, biochemistry, pathology, physiology, surgery. AYUSH-trained doctors are allowed to prescribe conventional medicines, but are expected to do so only in emergencies. Conventional medical training in India, by contrast, does not include the theory or practice of AYUSH. There is a theoretical proscription against MBBS doctors dispensing AYUSH remedies, although in practice, because of cost and demand, they often do. For day-to-day health problems, up to seventy per cent of Indians consult an AYUSH practitioner, not all of whom are licensed. There are a large number of 'fake doctors' who dispense pharmaceutical medicines: antibiotics, vitamin injections, steroids, but who have no training or qualifications at all.

India's healthcare system provides its citizens with enormous, if financially constrained, choice. In a country of twenty-two official languages and hundreds of dialects it is not surprising that there also exists a vast number of approaches to disease and its prevention. There are several non-AYUSH, non-biomedical traditions – folk, spiritual, herbal or ritual – whose practice remains ungoverned by the Ministry of Health despite the fact that they serve millions of people on a daily basis.

It is a hard truth that there are nowhere near enough trained health professionals to look after the sick among the country's 1.28 billion people, with MBBS doctor-to-patient ratios in rural areas, where seventy per cent of India's population live, reportedly as high as 100,000 to one, depending on the specialty in question. An additional problem is brain drain: many Indian doctors I spoke to, both in India and in other parts of the world, told me that the MBBS syllabus, its texts and its focus, seemed to concentrate on preparing young Indian doctors to work abroad, and less so on diseases they are likely to encounter in their home country. India is already the world's largest exporter of doctors, with about 47,000 currently practising in the United States and about 25,000 in the United Kingdom. On top of all this, for far too many, the cost of conventional medical treatment for common health problems is prohibitive and the distribution of drugs and the execution of public health programmes can face massive bureaucratic and logistical hurdles.

AYUSH, which has a better distribution of doctors in rural areas, offers partial solutions to some of these challenges. However, there is a limit to what AYUSH practitioners can achieve without additional training. Patients who use AYUSH out of choice or necessity do so for primary medical care, or to manage chronic conditions for which mainstream medicine offers no satisfactory alternative. For those with access to it, Western medicine is still the only option for conditions that require surgery or emergency intervention.

Meanwhile, in a public health service already short of staff, many institutions' 'full-time' doctors spend an untenable amount of time occupied with private patients. As will become evident during the course of this book, the lack of doctors can mean more than deprivation of healthcare, the vacuum filled too often by unqualified practitioners with access to potentially lethal medicines or scalpels, or spiritual healers wielding hot irons – sometimes with fatal consequences. Within private hospitals, some state-funded basic healthcare is available, but there are reports that those subsidised services are being withheld or misused.

In 2013 India ranked sixth in the Billionaire Census, registering more billionaires than Hong Kong, France, Saudi Arabia and Switzerland. For the country's rich (and super rich), and for the 300-million-strong middle class whose wealth is growing with the nation's, there are private hospitals. Exceptional hospitals. And plenty of them, in which those who can afford it receive world-class care as well as nips, tucks, Botox and skin whitening: aesthetic corrections involving invasive surgeries or procedures that can be done in the space of a lunch break. Though not so long ago seen as vain and unnecessary, beautifying India, one facial filler at a time, is now big business. Yet India's majority group

– the poor – remain excluded from even good basic medical care in conventional settings.

Studies of out-of-pocket spend on medical care in India show that people spend up to 100 per cent of their income on healthcare, particularly for chronic conditions. They also sell property in 'crisis financing' medical treatment for themselves or family members. For these reasons, the treatment of disease is plunging people into poverty, not pulling them out. In the absence of an adequate universal health insurance scheme, individual spending power remains key to healthcare access. And what of government investment? India spends less than one per cent of its gross domestic product (GDP) on healthcare, a proportion which is among the lowest in the world. Despite the country's phenomenal growth, its free healthcare compares very badly with other rapidly developing nations: Brazil, China, neighbouring Bangladesh – even Afghanistan. It is heartening that in 2015 India's prime minister, Narendra Modi, announced plans to double health expenditure to two per cent of GDP over the next five years, and in 2017, his government's Finance Minister Arun Jaitley presented ambitious action plans for improving health or ameliorating disease, including the creation of new public medical institutes of excellence and the scaling up and strengthening of medical education and training across the country.

But, even with these intended budgetary increases and efforts, India will still continue to spend less on the health of its population per capita and percentage of GDP than most other countries in the world. As it stands, India's government-subsidised urban and rural hospitals remain underfunded to the point of collapse, resulting in inadequately resourced and staffed state-sector hospitals attempting to cater for the nearly 250 million of India's rural population and 80 million city dwellers who live below the poverty line.

Given India's manifest challenges, it might seem absurd

that the country should pour money into backing unproven alternative treatments. Few Unani and Ayurveda remedies have been tested using the global 'randomised controlled clinical trial' standard and diagnoses are based on concepts like 'temperaments' (respectively, the four humours or three *doshas*) – a concept that Western medicine has not subscribed to for several hundred years. Plant- and animal-derived ingredients are used in their formulations, which is also true of an extensive list of modern drugs, and the recipes developed by old medical families over the centuries are secrets as closely guarded by AYUSH practitioners as the computer databases of Big Pharma. Such secrecy prevents the testing by the wider medical community of claims that AYUSH remedies have succeeded where scientific medicine has failed. Scientific medicine is supposed to improve by being exposed to criticism and testing – it may not always happen, but the principle still stands. By comparison, homoeopathy and naturopathy opt for a more mystical approach and their effects thought to be psychosomatic (although mainstream medicine may also rely to some degree on the placebo effect).

Why, then, is the Indian government so willing to embrace such esoteric alternatives? That was one of the questions I set out to explore in this book and, while writing it, I realised that the situation in India was far more complex than I had imagined. Though the science mattered both to me and to many of the medics I interviewed, for others compelling evidence had many avatars – from the heavily computed to the anecdotal to the entirely absent. Though there have been multiple attempts to root out 'unscientific' AYUSH medicine in India, it continues to flourish, sustained by word of mouth, accessibility and even recently a process of 'reorientalisation'. Ayurveda in particular has benefited from the latter, a process by which traditions of the East, becoming popular in the West, are re-exported to their countries of origin as an aspirational, glamorous choice.

But despite all these challenges, the story of Indian healthcare is one not solely of inequality and deprivation, but also of innovation, hope and passionate individuals who have moved heaven and earth to find solutions. Many of the initiatives I encountered – from Devi Shetty's chain of cardiac centres, which treat the poor for free, to the pioneering research project run by Pawan Sinha, which restores the sight of blind children – began as philanthropic initiatives of forceful individuals prepared to engage with Indian bureaucracy.

Some policy makers and local governments are more open to advice (and capable of implementing it) than others. Doctors Rani and Abhay Bang and their team in the Gadchiroli jungle, for example, created a health and research camp in response to the dire medical need of the local and tribal community. Their computer scientists and statisticians work in a hut in the centre of a campus built on family land bought with family funds. As well as developing public health programmes, their team of doctors also want to make sure that they are effective and efficient. Their work has influenced health policy both in India and across the world. It illustrates what can happen when the best doctors go to the places they are needed the most, though the pay is low and the conditions hard. The Bangs also study non-communicable disease – stroke, high blood pressure and diabetes in the tribal population – conditions more usually associated with overstressed, underexercised, overindulged city-dwellers rather than thin, active people who live close to the land. Their work shows that events and innovations in India have implications for the rest of the world: at a time when fewer of us are dying from infection, and instead living longer with debilitating, chronic 'lifestyle' diseases, the results of work like this are increasingly relevant.

So many others in these pages have had the courage, foresight, or at times even the folly to challenge a system whose opacity and complexity would defeat many, their persistence rewarded with support and funding from both individuals and international organisations. The scientist in my final chapter, Professor Pawan Sinha, for one, remains philosophical about the inherent difficulties. When I asked him about the challenges of working with the visually impaired in the country with the most blind people in the world, he said, quoting Khalil Gibran, 'When you set out to do something good, the energy of the universe aligns to assist you.'

Despite the work of these many inspirational individuals, there remains a long way to go before the ambition of that first government of modern India – state-supported healthcare for all – is realised. But if India is to achieve its full potential, it is a goal that remains vital: in one of the greatest nations on earth, the provision of world-class healthcare for all should be a major plank of government policy, not about philanthropy or ethics, or dependent on the goodwill of pioneering individuals. As an NHS colleague in London said to me – there is actually a strong economic case to be made as well. It is quite simply economic folly for a country to sacrifice its largest resource – its people – to ill health, poor nutrition and inadequate medical education.

Though I spent a good part of my childhood in India, hold an OCI (Overseas Citizen of India) card and was born to an Indian mother raised in Delhi and a Trinidadian father whose own father was taken into British indentured service from Uttar Pradesh, the stories in this book are still based on the observations of an outsider (though I think I have come to the conclusion that everyone is an outsider to some part of their own country, and even within their own cities). After completing my interviews for this book's final chapter, heavy-hearted to be leaving, I thought of something surgeon Dr Umang Mathur told me as I left the Dr Shroff Charity Eye Hospital in Delhi: 'India is everything they say it is,' he said, 'and nothing.'

Still, with an outsider's eyes, even in a familiar landscape, sometimes you find the most wonderful stories in unexpected places. And so, ultimately, this is a book about how people in India approach health. It places centre stage stories of Indians in the business of healing – from the forefront of cutting-edge medical science to traditional street-corner pharmacies dealing with all manner of diseases by all manner of means – all hoping to deliver a cure. In researching it, I have spent time with healers and with patients, finding out who they turn to and why. The projects I have covered and doctors I interviewed were chosen for a variety of reasons. Some were pioneers in their fields; others attracted celebrity clientele. Several have been powerful catalysts for change, or have long family histories of medical practice. Yet others are passionate folk practitioners who fuse ancient tradition with modern technology, or command vast numbers of patients who place their trust in them despite knowing little about the treatment they receive.

My aim was to allow characters and their stories to speak for themselves, vibrant snapshots of health and disease – both inside a rapidly changing nation and in the work of its diaspora, who have long comprised a disproportionately large percentage of doctors and scientists across the world.

Detailing the entire breadth and diversity of the practice of medicine in India is clearly beyond the scope of any single volume. For every individual research centre or hospital whose story I relate, there are hundreds of others whose narrative remains to be told. India has a long history of iconic, brilliant scientific and medical minds. Its interaction with the wider world, in the provision of knowledge, doctors or scientific or scholarly exchange, go back millennia. The archaeology of the sub-continent is increasingly uncovering Indian innovation, reaching far into its prehistory, and so there are an almost uncapturable number of tales to tell. I would encourage everyone to continue to explore, engage and collect the wisdom and wealth of human story this great country affords. Within the chapters that follow, my aim was to capture and curate a selection of stories that I found to reflect the experience of people from different socio-economic groups, from the educated to the illiterate, cities to forests, superstition to hard science. In India's rapidly changing landscape, any snapshot of 'now' is destined soon to become a mere record of practices, some of which, in just a few years' time, may well be obsolete. The stories told here move between rural and urban settings, from healing traditions rooted in India's religious, royal and colonial past to its twenty-first-century innovations. From neuroscience to jungle berries, ancient formulae to e-health, royal wrestlers to pioneering heart surgery, these are tales about medicine in India – as complex, vibrant, inspiring and bewildering as the country itself.

1

Depressed in Dharavi

WHERE '60-FEET ROAD' rises over the rail tracks, a short bridge loaded with abandoned heavy building materials and concrete mixers is a conduit to a part of Mumbai that its casual visitors – and many locals – would struggle to identify with. It's not that the slums of India's most glamorous city are invisible. Brought to the world's attention by the film *Slumdog Millionaire*, Mumbai's vast shanty towns envelope its international airport, so that the only way to be personally oblivious to the sea of blue tarpaulin or galvanized roofs is to land into the city by night.

ON THE GROUND, ask to be taken to Dharavi and a unidirectional shake of taxi drivers' heads will swiftly dismiss you. The driver who finally agreed to take me – for around three times the correct fare – compensated by doubling up as a tour guide. 'Dharavi is bigger than all slums,' he offered in Hindi, as we were held up in traffic next to a giant concrete mixer. 'Do you mean the biggest in Mumbai?' I saw a broad smile flash in the rear-view mirror. Taking a hand off the steering wheel, finger pointed upwards in a gesture of proclamation, there was an irony in his proud pronouncement that we were entering not just the largest slum in the city, but the largest in all Asia. At 535 acres and with a population of over 700,000, Mumbai's Dharavi is second only to the Neza-Chalco-Itza mega-slum in Mexico City.

Located in the heart of a city in which rents are on a par with New York and London, the slum's real-estate value is substantial. But towards 60-Feet Road, the Subways, Tata-allianced Starbucks, indie cafés and boutiques that are now familiar sights in the fashionable city disappear. There is a branch of Domino's Pizza just outside of Dharavi's borders, but they refuse to deliver there. En route from the airport you will find only one ATM, a stark contrast with their availability in other parts of Mumbai and a move by India's HDFC bank to capitalise on offering accounts to the many with little.

Along 60-Feet Road, English writing on signs and shop fronts suddenly, and almost completely, gives way to Hindi. Sometimes, on top of the makeshift roofs of the shanties lining the littered, sewage-filled waterways, you can make out large English print. To keep the monsoon at bay, a lucky few residents have acquired huge rectangles of tarpaulin that in a former life were election posters or adverts for new Mumbai luxury developments. The larger than life-sized photographs of politicians staring skyward create an inadvertent satire, as do the luxury property slogans they sport: *Have it all and save up to 72 lakh* (£70,000); *Serenity and blissful living*. Other than these, the only English in evidence over the bridge is an ALFA BOYZ gang tag sprayed onto a dirty concrete wall (possible competitors, I later learn, to the SlumGods, Dharavi's home-grown gang of breakdancing b-boys); and the words 'Praise the Lord', writ large on the windscreen of an old ambulance parked outside my destination.

Officially 'The Urban Health Centre in Dharavi', Chota Sion Hospital was built in 1980 as the government of Maharashtra State (of which Mumbai is the capital) began building tower blocks to rehouse Dharavi's early inhabitants and curb the slum's spread. Some of the first of these now blackened and dour blocks are directly opposite the hospital, designated *chota* (small) in deference to the main, fully equipped municipal Sion Hospital complex a few miles away. For a time, Chota Sion was set up to serve mainly the women and children of the slum, but it is now home to a strong team of social workers, an HIV/AIDS clinic, a vaccination centre and general wards. Because many husbands were reluctant to wear condoms, one of its most popular operations used to be voluntary female sterilisation, but today only minor surgery takes place here. Despite this, Chota Sion sits at the heart of Dharavi's community healthcare – both physical and mental.

Painted baby pink at some point in the distant past, the hospital's five storeys tower above the mass of shops and homes that surround it. As I stood at the main entrance, the smell of disinfectant and surgical spirit was nearly as strong as the sense of foreboding. It reminded me of a few war-torn and emptied buildings I had seen in Kabul, though this one, by contrast, was by no means abandoned. Doctors and patients went about their business, paying its state of disrepair no mind.

A guard directed me down a long corridor, past rooms where babies sat on their mothers' laps having their shots, or outpatients waited for check-ups. The busy STD clinic was decorated with a large drawing of a cartoon condom with arms, legs and a very happy face. I was surprised to see a lean white cat stride confidently along the corridor towards me, mewing loudly and looking quite at home as it passed the extensive lines of people sitting on the benches along its length, waiting to be seen. Much like the Domino's delivery team, it seemed that Mumbai's medical staff were also reluctant to serve Dharavi.

I made my way to the back of the building, which, apart from the wildlife, had an abandoned feel. On its main staircase, chipped cream paint and plaster had collected liberally along the edges of each step. A glance up the stairwell to the top of the building revealed thick red smears streaking the walls: not dried blood but the accumulation of years of betel nut-tinged spittle discharged from every floor, staining even the signs in place to forbid the practice.

To the right of the staircase I found the rear entrance to the hospital. A covered walkway cut through an open courtyard to a drive where a couple of atmospherically ancient ambulances were parked. It offered incoming patients some protection from the more vertical deluges of the multidirectional monsoon rains, as well as providing a waiting area for those who had come to approach Sabawa, the Goddess Oracle who sits for most of the day outside the hospital's courtyard shrine.

When I first saw her, Sabawa was holding court with a few devotees, her son, grandson and the men who had arrived that day with bamboo scaffolding to prepare the shrine for its annual festivity which would see the courtyard turned into a bloodbath. Her ample haunches were propped comfortably on a low wall; her retinue stood or sat on the floor around her. Their conversation paused as we *namasted*. There was something generally formidable about Sabawa, both in the powerful charisma she exuded and in her appearance – her dark, almost doll-like face adorned with a generous smile, two silver nose-rings and a too-large red circle on her forehead; her corpulent frame topped by black and grey mottled dreadlocks that tumbled nearly to her thighs. She was wrapped in a dark green sari, a colour sacred to the Goddess Kali and auspicious for married women; she'd covered her arms nearly to the elbows in green glass bangles too. Despite her girth, she looked nowhere near her seventy years.

And yet she had good reason not to look as well as she did because, thirty-two years ago, Sabawa, it was said, had inexplicably fallen ill and died.

Her son Rayvan told me this as nonchalantly as if he were giving directions. I asked him to repeat what he had said, just to make certain I had understood correctly. At first, when he told me his mother had died at the age of thirty-eight, I imagined that Sabawa had unofficially adopted him. But that was not at all what he meant.

Rayvan, with whom she had been pregnant at the time of her death, was Sabawa's youngest son, and when she was nearly to term she started experiencing strange and violent movements in her abdomen. Neighbours said that she had become possessed – that a *devi* (goddess) had entered her body. Like its gods, the goddesses of the Hindu pantheon often take on different avatars to become the spouses of their opposite-sex counterparts. This goddess – known as Kali, or Durga in her major incarnations – is the *shakti* (power) to the destroyer god Shiva, a forceful yin to his yang. Though a mother to the sons of gods and possessing the ability to be compassionate, she is no demure Mary nor bejewelled Lakshmi. Kali/Durga brings powerful, vengeful justice to the world.

The infiltration of this *devi*, or *bhoot* (ghost), into a person – usually a woman or a girl – is widely used across India to account for a range of symptoms that might otherwise be explained as depression, anxiety, epilepsy, malaise, rebelliousness or any number of psychiatric conditions. The treatments for possession can be incredibly brutal, and often extreme violence is inflicted on victims. Beatings and torture (including burning or rubbing chilli powder on the skin) are commonplace among believers. Sabawa was no exception, but the multiple hot irons that branded her stomach with circular burns did not cure her.

'After my mother died,' Rayvan continued, 'the community tied her hands and feet and wanted to take her body.' Sabawa's mother, distraught, prayed to an image of the goddess she kept at home and the next day announced to the community that the *devi* had spoken to her, warning that if they touched Sabawa's body they would all die. The goddess wanted this girl to care for her shrine and demanded blood. To bring Sabawa and her unborn child back from the beyond, two pregnant goats were to be slaughtered, their wombs opened and their unborn kids removed and sacrificed.

'It started with two, but now there are one hundred and fifty goats offered every year. Hindus, Muslims, everyone comes, it doesn't matter, they all come.' Rayvan beamed. His enthusiasm was understandable, as without the goddess's intervention, neither he nor Sabawa would have been there that day to tell me the story of the events that very nearly cost them both their lives.

It was sad to imagine what the young Sabawa and her family must have gone through during those difficult days. The cause of her convulsions and collapse (or possible coma) is difficult to guess at – even today, many women across India never have a thorough medical check-up during their pregnancies. Sabawa might have had epilepsy, or eclampsia seizures – symptoms which can worsen in the later stages of pregnancy. Or less scientifically, and perhaps more sinister, accusations of possession can sometimes be a cover for simply getting rid of a person, in a vendetta, for example, or a witch-hunt. Whatever the cause, Sabawa was lucky to have recovered, an outcome the family ascribes entirely to divine intervention. In those early days in that slum, as still in many parts of India, the lack of access to appropriate medical care means that the intervention of spiritual healers can seem like the only recourse, sometimes with fatal consequences.

Since her personal triumph over disease and desperation, the faith of Sabawa and her sons in the *devi* has been intense. The *devis* whose statues filled that shrine (no more than the size of a shower cubicle) seemed even more so. Her devotees, who were often also Chota Sion patients, came every day to make offerings. They brought the green glass bangles and marigolds that laced their way around the dome of the shrine; they came to ask for healing or offer thanks for prayers granted. But more than that, they came to hear the goddess speak through Sabawa's voice, and for that they also brought goats and chickens to be sacrificed (and, rumour has it, not insubstantial offerings of gold).

'When the goat is brought for sacrifice I ask the *devi* whether she accepts the sacrifice or not. If I see the goat trembling it is the sign of *devi*'s acceptance, it is a sign to kill her for the sacrifice.'

Sabawa says she demands no sacrificial offerings or valuables, but her devotees bring them anyway. The green glass bangles she welcomes, and the flowers are useful decoration for both the goddesses and her oracle's stone, which she asks people to touch and make a wish.

'It's just a stone,' Rayvan told me. He pointed to a rubble-strewn area across the fence, around two metres away. 'Look there, my mother just picked it up from the other side of the courtyard. My mother could use any stone, the goddess still speaks.'

It wasn't really just any stone: placed in front of the goddesses, directly in her eye-line, was a rock about fifty centimetres in length and twenty-five wide. Its edges were slightly jagged, as was its underside, so that it wasn't entirely stable. When Sabawa sat before it and put her petitioners' questions to the goddess, the rock would become the instrument of her voice.

'When the answer is yes, stone will move to the right; if it is a no, the stone swings left,' he explained. Rayvan bent down and pushed it to one side and then the other. 'See, see how heavy it is … it cannot move on its own.'

As he walked off, I tried it too. It didn't even budge. 'It is incredibly heavy,' I agreed.

'Yes. And when the goddess gets angry, the stone moves fast, forward towards the shrine, like this!' The push of Rayvan's upturned hands indicated a violent movement and I imagined a great crash against the front wall of the shrine.

I hurried after him. 'Does she get angry often? Why would she get angry?'

I knew that Kali and her various alter egos were no soft

touch. While Lakshmi sits on a lotus and radiates loveliness and light, Kali and Durga are popularly depicted with semi-crazed eyes and hair, wearing garlands of human skulls, holding swords dripping with blood, or mounted on large predatory animals. When the goddess entranced Sabawa, she too danced wildly, energetically, with the vigour of a far younger woman. 'Even just after she had undergone a major heart operation in her late sixties,' said Rayvan.

'Too many questions,' he went on. I stayed silent. 'When there are too many people at the shrine asking the goddess questions,' he clarified, 'it's too much. The goddess gets tired. She gets angry.'

Kali, the goddess Rayvan had been referring to, was personified in a stone statue, not more than thirty centimetres in height, that was housed in the shrine. Had it not been for Kali's rage, the Chota Sion shrine would never have existed. It had not been built for the hospital, as many locals and staff believe; in fact, it appears to have been a sacred site for at least 500 years, and the hospital must therefore have been built around it.

Today Dharavi, like much of Mumbai, seems as though it has always been solid ground, but a substantial part of the coastal city was dredged from marshland by impoverished migrants. Within living memory, many parts of the now crowded metropolis were countryside, largely unchanged for hundreds of years, and when the statue of the terrible Kali was originally unearthed, what would one day be 60-Feet Road was still farmland. A farmer ploughing his field had dug up what turned out to be the image of Sabawa's goddess. It was reminiscent of the famous twelfth-century Janganatha statues of Puri – wide-eyed, cartoon-like, naive – though this was not to be her personality. Unfortunately, the statue was damaged by the farmer's plough, and the landowner's carelessness was to cost him dear. His entire family died mysteriously, and he built the shrine in an effort to secure his absolution.

No one could say exactly when this had happened, but Rayvan believed it was in the fourteenth century because the goddess came to him in a dream one night and told him so. When Chota Sion was being constructed, the builders unwisely destroyed the ancient shrine. The goddess's revenge was no slower in the 1980s than it had been in the 1300s: soon labourers started falling unconscious and unexplained calamities befell both patients and staff. The worker who had demolished it was found with an iron rod through him, vomiting blood. The shrine was swiftly reinstated and a courtyard created where there had been a hospital wing on the blueprint.

Through her oracle Sabawa, this powerful and avenging goddess continues to draw Dharavi's women to her: women who are in abusive marriages, women who, for whatever reason, are considered by their families to be mad. 'The *devi* normally enters people when they are having many problems,' Rayvan said. Possession and a distressed state of mind are inevitably linked. Sadly, as I would later learn, many Mumbai psychiatrists are unwilling to link the same distress to a more prosaic cause: the domestic abuse suffered by Dharavi's women.

Compounding this, there is no psychiatric department at Chota Sion. This situation is by no means unusual.

World Health Organisation data reports that there are only 43 mental hospitals with in-patient care in the country; for every 100,000 people, there are only two hospital beds reserved for mental health. Though many parents in the country and among its diaspora populations hope their children will grow up to be doctors, in India psychiatrists are not held in particularly high esteem. It is estimated that there are only between 3,500 and 5,000 psychiatrists in the entire country, a number which equates to one doctor to 200,000–300,000 people. At the main Sion Hospital (less well known by its official name, Lokmanya Tilak Municipal General Hospital) victims of domestic violence – generally women – are typically treated for injuries, but not for the wider issues involving emotional or psychiatric fallout because the resources for this are in short supply. To fill the gap between the way Western medicine separates body and mind, patients often consult a *baba* (holy man) to get rid of the *bhoot*, but Sabawa believes they are charlatans who take money in exchange for false promises or useless treatments. She is very clear that when patients come to her for help, she first asks them if they have already been to see the psychiatrists at Sion. She asks whether they had been given medicine and whether they have taken it. She will agree to intercede 'Only if nothing else has helped. Then, it is the work of the *devi*.'

In the traditional and folk forms of medicine practised in India, diseases of the body are intricately linked to the condition of the mind, and perhaps also to the idea of a soul. The lack of dissonance in many of those who came to Chota Sion was fascinating – patients were perfectly at ease making an offering to the *devi* as they passed the shrine en route to their medical appointments inside the building. They had come to be healed, by whatever means.

This sometimes resulted in clashes between the *devi*'s courtyard representatives and the hospital medics over the best way to treat their devotees-patients. During one of Sabawa's rare departures from the shrine, Shankar, the thirty-four-year-old priest-in-training, thought it best to leave a young woman, who had collapsed while waiting in the covered walkway, rolling about the paving slabs in convulsions. Though Shankar had not expected the goddess to jump into action in his mistress's absence, it seemed entirely reasonable to him that she had chosen to take over this young woman's body. After all, she had come for divine intervention and Kali Maata was not one to disappoint. However, the truth was that the young woman had been waiting not to consult the oracle, but for her father, who was inside collecting his daughter's epilepsy medication having left her sitting comfortably on the low wall that bordered the shrine.

Three floors higher, on a wing of Chota Sion that was bisected by the red-stained stairwell, Western medicine ruled unopposed. The back half of the wing was an L-shaped women's ward and, much like the staircase, its brutalist space had a long-forgotten quality. Rows of vintage, uncurtained metal-framed beds stood close together policed by severe nurses in old-fashioned, starch-stiffened dresses with navy epaulettes and matching wimples. Infants lay with their mothers on some of the beds; husbands, brothers, fathers sat in the waiting area outside.

Walking across the hall was like moving forward four decades. I stepped into a corridor of neatly partitioned offices, where smart young women in *kurti* tops and jeans were busy at their phones or computers: some developing apps, I later discovered, using open source data and GPS to help women in the slums map violence with their phones. Preventing violence, gender inequality and its consequences – depression, anxiety, addiction, disease and disability – was the business of Nayreen Daruwala, a doctor of social psychology who had specialised in mental health. Her office was one of four cubicles which made up the offices of SNEHA: the Society for Nutrition, Education & Health Action, set up nineteen years after Dharavi's hospital with the aim of reducing maternal and newborn mortality, malnutrition and domestic violence.

The room was large, white and sparse, furnished only with a desk, her laptop, a mobile phone, four plastic chairs and a ceiling fan that was never silent. The folders shelved in a small built-in cupboard made her office a hub of interaction, with a regular influx of colleagues fishing out files, raising questions and engaging in project discussions with Nayreen, whose warmth and energy were almost palpable. Either side of the filing cupboard, windows framed sections of the vast spread of tightly packed, monsoon-sodden tarpaulin-covered houses down below, giving a powerful sense of being entirely enclosed by the slum. Through the windows, damp breezes brought the smell of rain and periodic refrains of *Allahhu akbar* from Dharavi's muezzins below.

I asked Nayreen what she made of the goings-on in the hospital shrine below.

'After the hospital rebuilt the shrine, people started considering Sabawa to be pious and asked her to help them out in difficult situations by praying to the goddess – they approach her in difficult situations, they make offerings of goats as a sacrifice to alleviate problems in their lives and appease the *devi*. People resort to all sorts of things in Dharavi – there are healers for jaundice, skin, mental health, venereal disease, blindness; there are bone-setters. Dharavi is a mini India, it's amazing how they blend over here.'

The slum had certainly been a magnet for economic migrants from the countryside. Nayreen explained the difficulties facing farmers in making even a small profit or repaying loans. Among farmers in India, suicide rates are shocking. But an income was not the only reason people came. 'Healthcare in Mumbai is actually quite good – in fact there are people who come to Dharavi especially to get treatment,' Nayreen continued. 'Some of them may already have had family here, but while they waited six months to be seen, or while they or their parents or wives or children continued their treatment, they became settled. They work here, their kids start going to school, they stay. On the other hand, some people have a distrust of medicines and hospitals,' she continued. 'They say, "I'm not *mad*." They think they get ill because someone "put something on them". If women are in anxiety or depression, they'll say, "She's got the devil in her – when it leaves, she'll be fine," or when they have an attack, they'll go to a *baba*. They'll be fine for a while, but then come again to Chota Sion.'

The gender-based violence project that she heads came about when a neonatal doctor called Armida Fernandes noted that many of her patients were talking about the violence they faced at home. She was trying to save mothers in labour and the lives of their new babies, but realised that nothing was being done to protect their health once they left the hospital. Together Armida and Nayreen began approaching every doctor at Chota Sion, asking that they refer anyone showing signs of domestic violence for psychological intervention. The assessment of the mental health of women suffering abuse was something that had never before been offered to Mumbai's poorest migrant families.

It was slow to get off the ground, with women reluctant to consider counselling. 'They'd say, "I don't need treatment, give me money for my daughter's education instead,"' Nayreen recalled. It came as no surprise. Physical violence, particularly towards wives, is accepted as normal. 'Many women say things like, "He was right to beat me, I didn't put enough salt in the food," or the husband's parents ask their son, "Why are you treating her so nicely? You should beat her." It's accepted by men and women, it's the husband's right.'

Throughout 2001, Nayreen recorded intervention in only seventy-eight cases; they now have a database of 4,000, ninety per cent of whom are residents of Dharavi. 'I've seen women come in with all kinds of conditions – terrible head injuries, broken noses. But because the centre has become more popular, we see women coming earlier.'

In Dharavi, one-brick partition walls divide the crush of tiny houses. These rows of homes have front doors that face each other across narrow alleys – gully streets in which people must almost press against each other to pass. Here, privacy is rare and community is key. It was the power of word of mouth – *gupshup*, chit-chat, the intervention of mothers, elder sisters, aunts – that saw SNEHA's initiative snowball. Through aligning with these intimate lines of communication, Nayreen's fifteen years building the counselling centre at Chota Sion have given her an encyclopaedia of stories ranging from the inspiring to the weird and the simply terrifying. There was the tale of the woman who dipped a piece of paper into her husband's tea every morning to cast a spell on him to curb his infidelity. It was her way of taking control in a world where women have little. More alarmingly, the soothsayers who 'prescribe' these chits of magic paper sometimes also infuse them with herbal poisons, for extra potency.

Then there was the story of one of Nayreen's colleagues, Sitaram, and the exorcism performed on his wife after a seven-day prayer session in the local Presbyterian church. 'But Sitaram is a Hindu name,' I said, confused. Nayreen smiled. 'No one can explain how his wife got better. There must be an explanation, but it seems like a miracle – she was very severely ill. You should ask him about it.'

When I found Sitaram, he was in an arts centre that Nayreen and colleagues had set up. Finding space for an art gallery in Dharavi had been a costly challenge, but inside Colour Box the work of local women was being arranged for the Dharavi Biennale – the world's only Biennale hosted in a slum. The art they had made – textiles, furniture, paintings with themes of family, martial discord, rape, dreams of homes that were safe and salubrious for their children – functioned as therapy, as well as developing vocational skills and for earning an income for the artists. The facade of the narrow rented building – which had once been crumbling plaster and exposed brick – had already been painted with the project's colourful logo, a quadrant containing a heart, an eye, a cross and the symbol for infinity, symbolising health, art and recycling. Like the tarpaulins from luxury apartment builds, in Dharavi, everything became something else.

Outside Colour Box, Sitaram greeted me jovially, chatting as we walked back to Chota Sion and periodically shielding me from the chaotic rush of vehicles which paid pedestrians no heed. He was the kind of person anyone would take an instant liking to: friendly, funny – with a delightful grin that lifted up his neat moustache when it appeared. As he negotiated the feinting umbrellas and found us footholds along the main road, which was rapidly filling with water, he told me how his wife, who had been diagnosed with multidrug-resistant tuberculosis and given months to live, had woken up one morning speaking in tongues. Specifically, in Tamil, a south Indian language that she had no previous knowledge of or exposure to. Sitaram had been born into a Hindu family from a rural Maharashtra village, raised in Dharavi and later became a convert to Christianity. Much as the patients who saw no conflict in making offerings at Sabawa's shrine en route to accessing modern medicine for the problems that ailed them, Sitaram seemed to be relating a similar underlying narrative in which, in seeking a cure, the lines between the spiritual and the physical were blurred. When doctors were unable to effectively treat his wife's tuberculosis, she both continued drug treatment and turned to the Christian church – and later the Hindu temple – in the hope of being healed. Though bearing parallels to *devi* possession, speaking in tongues seemed like a particularly 'Christian' phenomenon, for which Sitaram naturally turned to a Dharavi church.

'We are from a village in Maharashtra; Varsha, my wife, spoke only Marathi,' Sitaram told me.

'So how did you end up at the church? Is your family Christian?' I asked.

'My family all converted. I did too. I was happy to.' He smiled his jolly smile. 'I like Jesus. We took my wife to the church and the priests sat in a circle around her and prayed. She kept talking in Tamil, but after seven days, she stopped. She was healed.'

'And what about the tuberculosis?' I asked.

'For that, there was nothing we could do. Her lungs

seemed entirely damaged. The medicines were not working. I sent her back to the village for a while with the children – I had to work but I thought she would be much more relaxed there, it is less stressful, you see.'

I nodded.

'In the village she was taken to the temple. The *devi* is worshipped there, she was the goddess we prayed to before. In the temple, the villagers said prayers for her. Then the goddess spoke to one of the village women and she told us, "Your family has left your own gods, your own beliefs. Come back to the goddess and whatever is inside your wife will leave her." Varsha stayed in the temple. There they prayed over her and one day, her hair suddenly became wild like the goddess's. They told me the goddess had entered her and when she went back to normal, after the prayers had finished, she was better. The tuberculosis had gone.'

As we arrived at the gates to Chota Sion, I found myself partly attempting to calculate the probability of recovery from an apparent advanced state of lung damage and partly getting used to the divine modus operandi that Dharavi's residents seemed perfectly at ease with.

By the time SNEHA opened its doors in 1999, its clientele had long since become inured to cases of extreme violence to which both they and the police routinely turned a blind eye. Back in her third-floor office, rain still battering the tarpaulins below, Nayreen recalled to me her frustration at two early cases concerning the murder of young women. The first victim was the fourth wife of a man who set her on fire because she had brought no dowry. The second case was very similar, but in neither were there any witnesses willing to give evidence. Nayreen had told me of the strength of the community in Dharavi's mini-India. The bond between neighbours that provided fraternal support, but which could also become a wall of silence in the face of trouble, would become one of the greatest allies and obstacles to SNEHA's work.

And then another murder was reported. 'This time it was a twenty-one-year-old woman who had just got married. While she was walking home one day, two men followed her making lewd suggestions. When she ignored their catcalls, they said she had disrespected them. The next evening they and one of the men's wives came to her door and forced their way in, severely beat her, locked her in her house and then set it alight.'

As the recent reports of gang rape testify, violence against women in India remains a depressingly intractable problem today, not just in Dharavi but across socio-economic groups throughout the country. But for Nayreen, this historic burning drove home the fact that the circle of violence and mental illness among both women and men would require much more than counselling if it were ever to be broken. 'The whole community saw what was happening, but no one intervened – and afterwards, no one would talk. We had no clue what we were going to do. There were several other NGOs that could have helped gather evidence, but none did.'

While the badly burned victim fought for her life in hospital, Nayreen continued to work with police and the public prosecutor, trying to to build a case against those responsible.

'I was curious about why no one in such a tight-knit community was prepared to speak out about such a brutal and unprovoked murder of one of their own.' Nayreen ascribed it to a mixture of fear and the cultural acceptance, ingrained over centuries, that men had the right to assault women with impunity. Mothers often stay in abusive relationships only for the sake of their children, and sometimes blame them too: Nayreen has heard five-year-olds say that they feel it is their fault that their mothers suffer. The deep and lasting psychological damage of such cycles of violence is not difficult to imagine.

'It's the whole family unit – that case made me understand that traditional psychotherapy would not be possible,' she went on. The 'family unit' in Nayreen's terminology was far broader than immediate relations. It included those who held honorary titles of uncle or aunt (who could be anyone at all) and even close neighbours. All were invested in their community relationships, so any could be quite seriously affected. 'Slums are strong communities. When I began offering counselling sessions, the whole family would come – mother, sisters, neighbours. It became community counselling.'

The girl who had been attacked died from her burns, but she first rallied sufficiently to give a statement identifying her killers, who were subsequently gaoled for fourteen years.

Because of her involvement, Nayreen had become a target. 'One of the men swore that he would take revenge on me. I don't know what will happen. There are only a few years to go now until he's released. But he's had counselling in prison, he is not as violent as he was.'

Stoic as she is about the murderer's reformation, it would be a satisfying end to a sad, violent story if he were to emerge from his sentence a milder man. To change the trajectory of culturally accepted violence has always been the aim of Nayreen and her team. There are now ninety-two local women's groups with more than a thousand members, and counselling programmes at Chota Sion that both women and their husbands attend regularly.

In India today, the healthcare given to many women is ensnared in gender inequality. Under her perpetually whirring ceiling fan, Nayreen and her colleagues explained to me at length how differently men and women are treated when they become physically or mentally ill – barriers that can be erected both by the Indian healthcare system and by the people it is supposed to serve. Gauri, the coordinator for SNEHA's counselling centre, described to me how, in many Dharavi families, if a man is ill it's common practice to take him to hospital, while a woman in the same situation is just given a bottle of simple painkillers by her in-laws and stays at home. 'And worse,' she told me, 'depression – any kind of mental illness in women – is seen as grounds for divorce; a reason to abandon their wives with nothing, no support.'

'There was one couple referred to me,' said Nayreen. 'Both were HIV positive, but the husband blamed the wife, saying that she had given it to him. That wasn't true, it was quite the other way around. Anyway, as I told you, people in Dharavi will try everything, so the husband went to some untrained Ayurvedic doctor – at least the man claimed to be a doctor – who said he could cure the husband, but he was very expensive. Now the wife was pregnant with their second child at the time – their first child was also HIV positive – but when our doctors recommended a termination, the husband refused to give permission. The whole family was convinced it was her fault. They took away her first child and were treating him with whatever this self-proclaimed Ayurvedic doctor was charging them for. She was distraught. We intervened legally and the child was returned to her, but he did not survive. The husband also died. The good news is that she survived, and she has now remarried a man who is also HIV positive, so she has a family again. Her second child is free of HIV.'

'The same thing happens if a woman is depressed,' Gauri explained. 'Her in-laws will abandon her. If a doctor or counsellor diagnoses depression, the husband just says she's mad and leaves her. There was a depressed woman whose husband was schizophrenic and had erectile dysfunction and his family blamed it on her because they said she was mad. Her husband tried to use her illness as grounds for divorce.'

Fortunately, the Indian courts knew better. The judge told the woman's in-laws that they could not remove her from her home, that she was not 'mad' if she could get better with treatment and ordered that she should receive appropriate care that would improve her condition.

'The problem is,' Nayreen told me, 'women need sleep when they are on medication, but they are not allowed to rest. They are still expected to wake up early to do the cooking, the chores, so the husbands and in-laws see this "laziness" as justification for assault. There is no respite.'

Inside the maze of lanes and alleyways that formed the capillaries of the slum, I met three women who had experienced abandonment and abuse first hand and who now work with SNEHA to intervene and support others in the same situation. Their homes and their places of work were deep in the warren of lanes, and so that I was able to get there – and out again – Nayreen's colleague Bhaskar offered to show me the way.

Ankle-deep in filthy water made worse by the rapidly accumulating rains, I followed Bhaskar off 60-Feet Road and into another world. Past sweetshops and one-room barber salons, small vegetable stalls and video stores that became pornography cinemas by night, we entered through a lane flanking one of Dharavi's waterways. Liberally strewn with all manner of rubbish, the canal also served as a sewer. The slum's infrastructure facilitated this – some of the settlement's communal toilet cubicles were designed to protrude over the water. There was only room here to walk in single file. Bhaskar spoke little and walked fast and I struggled to navigate the uneven, submerged paving slabs to catch up with him in my sodden shoes. A small boy walking behind me was becoming increasingly irritated at my slowing him down, so that from behind me I could hear an unrelenting Hindi narrative describing my incompetence as he made several failed attempts to overtake. Eventually, as we turned off the canal way into the rows of tiny, brightly painted brick houses, I saw his spindly legs speed off into the distance. My young daughter was with us and I saw her look of utter desperation as she gave up trying to keep our umbrella open – though by no means large, it was wider than the lane between the houses.

As we came to what seemed to be a dead end, Bhaskar gestured left, inviting us to see the toilets. Six cubicles were laid out in a square, three either side of a small passage. At the end was a large hole in the wall that served as a window. It overlooked a swamp, a reminder of what the entire area was before it became Dharavi. It was bleak and wild and, had it not been heaped with still higher piles of rubbish than I had seen in other parts of the slum, it might even have been beautiful. Bhaskar explained how plans were afoot to seal the hole in the wall. 'These toilets are for women,' he explained. 'Boys know that and come here. They jump through this hole, grab the girls and take them out there – sometimes with their consent, other times not. It makes it a dangerous place for the women in the community.' It was a horrible thought, to imagine a girl abducted, molested and then abandoned in that stinking, muddy marsh.

A few steps on we arrived at a pastel-pink building which was home to Chandravati, a pretty, chubby woman in her late thirties who served as one of SNEHA's *sanghinis*, or female community workers. As I took off my soaking shoes before entering, her husband went to stand outside the front door. When I stepped in, I realised why. Her house, like all the houses in Dharavi, was a windowless, waterless, bathroomless ten-foot-square box and within it lived her entire family. Three of her seven children were lying on the floor as Chandravati attempted – unsuccessfully – to rouse them from their siesta to get them back to school for the afternoon. The room looked as though its primary use was as a kitchen, with various pots lining the shelves of one wall. On the opposite wall was a television and a narrow *charpoy* where she and her husband slept, though it was hard to see how they could both occupy it at the same time. She offered us a seat on its mattress and snapped one of her daughters into action to run out and buy us biscuits and soda to snack on as we talked.

'Don't the kids want to go to school?' I asked Chandravati, who was still cajoling the sleeping trio.

'My son is not so keen but my daughters are,' she told me. 'They like school ... but they don't want to go out in the rain.'

I didn't blame them.

'Ninety per cent of the kids here do go to school now,' Bhaskar explained. 'It's improved a lot. But once they get married they stop. They still marry young here, boys and girls. The boys work, the girls will be housewives.'

Just then, another of Chandravati's daughters, much too small for her seventeen years, appeared at the front door with a friend. She was dressed in a new ornate sari and jewellery. Her mother explained that she had recently been married, but that her new home was a long way away, albeit in a nicer neighbourhood. Now, there were only eight people in that beautifully kept little pink box. Though that must have offered some small relief, and Chandravati seemed very matter-of-fact about it, I thought the girl looked a little too young to have already left home and, despite her pride at having a daughter who had clearly married well, I could see her mother missed her. Still, at least she was away from the immediate danger of the toilets next door.

The danger posed by those toilets was what originally motivated Chandravati to volunteer with SNEHA. That and the reluctance of the municipal corporation to clean blocked drains, the problem of drug addiction among young men and the general harassment of women and girls in the community. She began intervening directly in cases of violence that the community reported or when she saw any girl being harassed by 'goons'. She and three other local women joined forces and became the Dharavi's 'vigilance inspectors'. Once, for example, when they heard that a boy had dragged a girl into the creek from the toilet and molested her, her team staked out the toilet until he eventually reappeared, whereupon they detained him and handed him over to the police. They also made sure that the police patrolled in the area regularly. What she and her colleagues had managed to achieve in an often lawless and dangerous place through sheer determination was impressive. But Chandravati was clear about what she still wanted to see happen in Dharavi. 'My dream,' she said, 'is to help empower women and girls to be courageous and live better lives. I want them to stop crying when they face violence and instead ask for help and support at the right time to free themselves from the situation.'

A community meeting was to be held that afternoon on the other side of the main canal, organised by two of Dharavi's other *sanghinis*, and I wanted to listen in. Stepping once again out into the narrow slum lanes, I turned to see her husband quietly head back into the house, now emptied of children and guests.

My daughter and I took an auto-rickshaw to get to the meeting – partly because of the unrelenting rain and partly because of Dharavi's immense sprawl. As we walked from the rickshaw back into the maze we passed one of the little temple squares – the only non-claustrophobic spaces among the dark narrow lanes – and arrived at the home of Bhanuben, another *sanghini*. This time there were fifteen local women in the sparsely furnished ten-foot square kitchen-cum-living room, sitting cross-legged and taking up almost the entire floor space. As we entered, wondering where we might sit, Bhanuben, a jovial but forceful woman in her mid-forties, dressed in a sari and sporting a large bindi; and fellow *sanghini* Shirin, a much younger woman draped in a black *hijab* and *jilbab*, welcomed us in as warmly as if the room was of palatial proportions. We folded our legs into the shape of the last visible pieces of painted concrete. Shirin stood nearby, leaning in to translate in case I missed any of the discussion.

By then, the talk that had paused when I entered was once again in full flow. It had come to Bhanuben's attention that there had been several child marriages – eleven- and twelve-year-olds. Had anyone else come across this? Many of the group chipped in – it was a matter of grave concern, for both boys and girls who were leaving school prematurely to raise families. What might be done about it?

The next point on the agenda was a deeply fascinating question that wouldn't have been given a second thought in those places where mothers arranged play dates and coffee mornings, but which felt distinctly out of place in Dharavi. 'What do you do for *yourselves*?' Bhanuben asked. 'What makes you happy? Is it singing, is it dancing? Do you spend some time on yourselves every day?' She spoke forcefully and seemingly from a well of experience, so that, as they were raised, she swiftly, skilfully and kindly put down every protestation or excuse from the women in the group.

'I do not have any time to do something for myself,' the young woman next to me said. 'I am always cooking, or looking after children, or my husband. Where is there time?' She laughed at Bhanuben's deliciously ridiculous idea.

The woman directly opposite me was far less cheerful. 'I have three children and I look after them on my own. One of them is ill. He has epilepsy. I cannot afford his medicine. I cannot find work.' It was true, jobs were difficult to come by and life was hand-to-mouth for all the women present. In state-run hospitals, a nominal charge of ten rupees (ten pence) is made for medications, but I knew from my conversations with Nayreen that even that small amount might present a choice between treatment or their children's next meal. I could see that 'me time' was the farthest thing from her mind.

'That is why we are meeting here,' Bhanuben said. 'There is support. Come to Chota Sion and tell SNEHA that you are needing that medicine. We will help you. There are twenty-four hours in a day. I am not asking you for all of them. I am asking you to take half an hour for yourself.

Half an hour a day to do what you enjoy. You can do that. Raise your hands if you will do that. What time of day will you make time? What will you do?'

A few tentative hands rose into the air, unsure, like weighted balloons ready to drop at a moment's notice. But the more hands that went up, the more other women were emboldened to join in until nearly everyone agreed to give it a try. 'When I was a girl I wanted to sing,' one of the group offered her pledge. 'I *really* wanted to learn, but my parents would not allow me. I was very angry at them. *That* is what I will do now, I can spend some time singing.' But at the back of the room, another of the women sat quietly. She looked melancholic, beyond sadness, her face devoid of expression, her eyes empty. It was the look of someone recently bereaved, though she has lost no one to death.

'My husband left,' she said. 'I have two children. Now my children do not listen to anything I say. They don't have jobs. I don't have a job or money ...' I could see it must have felt to her as though everything was conspiring against her, and it was a heaviness I deeply related to also, having always raised my daughter on my own. She looked defeated, but at least she spoke and was listened to. I watched as Bhanuben counselled her and the group around her offered support. There was not one woman there who couldn't relate to at least part of what she was experiencing. The absence of a husband through death or abandonment, or the presence of an abusive one, was evidently a burden most had in common.

Shirin, who had been translating for me, had also experienced this at first hand. Extremely eloquent and clearly very well educated, she had been forced to move out of the marital home with her children after her husband had remarried. Without support from the community group, she would not have had the courage to reclaim the space in her house and regain stability for her children. That was what made her want to do the same for other women who felt powerless, or were in the depths of depression. 'I am alert and keep my eyes open for women [in crisis], motivate them to ask for help. Abandoned women whose husbands have remarried; women and girls being harassed by the local boys. I am proud of myself to be a *sanghini*,' said Shirin. With Bhanuben, she encouraged women to attend meetings for emotional and social support and to train for skilled jobs.

When Bhanuben wasn't finding women in crisis, women in crisis were finding her. She would always answer a knock on her door, whatever the hour. Her social work came later in life, twenty-four years after she dropped out of school, aged twelve. She married at sixteen and then began working as a domestic cook, which provided her husband and in-laws with their only income. She always dreamed of studying again, but didn't know how to. Her husband's family was very conservative and in their community it was taboo for a woman to go out wearing even ankle jewellery, or even to wear it indoors if it could be seen by other male relatives.

When Bhanuben finally made the decision to do something for herself – as she encourages other women to do – she was ridiculed by the local council of elders. When the social work done by her team of women started to produce results, they were condemned by the men of the community and their husbands were openly taunted for 'not having control over their wives and letting them do such work'. But still her work continues. Bhanuben, a born leader, if not a force of nature, was adamant that it should. 'Joining SNEHA was like being reborn, and in the same way other women should also reinvent themselves.' Her community group now has over a hundred members who educate and support others in matters of violence and women's rights. The men of the local council who once ridiculed her now respect her. And many of those husbands who were abusive or addicts have also turned up for counselling at Chota Sion.

Back at the hospital, Nayreen Daruwala was cautiously pleased at the community's progress. 'It has snowballed; people are referred by family and friends. Counselling is slowly becoming part of the culture. Even some men in Dharavi who have had counselling are referring abused women and their abusers to the centre now.'

But there is still a long path to travel, and its direction is one that excites Nayreen. 'Mental health is *so* tied up with violence here. Psychiatrists in Mumbai won't accept this. They hold only a genetic and physiological viewpoint about mental health conditions.'

I found it incredible that Nayreen and her team were having a hard time getting psychiatrists in the main Sion Hospital to acknowledge a relationship between violence and the development of mental illness in women. Through SNEHA's recent interventions – creating the beginnings of a women's outpatient department and offering counselling services for survivors of violence – Nayreen still hopes to highlight this association to the medics.

Clearly, many of the women who will go to SNEHA's outpatient department for counselling will improve over time because of psychological therapies – the 160 *sanghinis* now serving Dharavi are evidence of that. 'Almost every woman we interact with have faced some form of violence, either in their homes or in the community,' Nayreen told me. Not all of them require psychiatric drug-based therapy, but by highlighting an association that most Indian psychiatrists do not currently acknowledge, the hope is that more women who need it will have access to medical help. This is also crucial to changing the culture of how women are treated both medically and socially. From in-laws dispensing tablets to psychiatrists who will not, changing that culture of second-rate treatment for women will mean getting an acknowledgement that women who are depressed in Dharavi are not just 'mad', or a write-off to be divorced or abandoned. It will be a recognition that violence and its psychological or psychiatric effects are no longer acceptable or invisible; that women can and will be treated, and in many cases not only improve but also themselves become powerful agents of change.

2

Bollywood Bodies

ACROSS THE BRIDGE over the Mithi River, a fifteen-minute drive west of Dharavi will take you past yet more expanses of temporary, tarpaulin-covered makeshift homes populated by families who cannot afford even to live in the mega-slum. In contrast, the Bandra Kurla Complex, a carefully planned quarter of Mumbai reminiscent of Seoul or Abu Dhabi, feels, as a colleague working in Dharavi described it, like entering 'an off-world, like in science-fiction books'. BKC, as it is popularly known, has wide roads, towering office buildings clad in mirrored glass, five-star hotels hosting pool parties, swanky pizza restaurants and the American Embassy, set behind metal fences more than three times the height of the average Indian.

Bandra Kurla is also home to the Asian Heart Hospital, a large, multi-speciality health complex built, like most of the surrounding neighbourhood, only a decade or so ago. Offering everything from robotic surgery to neurology, orthopaedic to dental and cosmetic surgery, it is the hospital equivalent of a luxury hotel.

I was there to meet Dr Satish Arolkar, serving president of the Indian Association of Plastic Surgeons and the man responsible for introducing India to liposuction and, back in the 1980s in the days before silicone implants, breast enhancement by fat graft. In the intervening years, Dr Arolkar would tell me, once Mumbai had overcome its initial qualms regarding the vanity and drastic nature of aesthetic surgery, it had forged ahead and never looked back.

Data from the International Society of Aesthetic Plastic Surgeons make it hard to disagree: India is certainly at the centre of a worldwide boom in cosmetic surgery. In 2011, out of the 15 million people who resorted to plastic surgery to enhance their looks, 466,231 were Indians. That puts India well within the world top ten by number for a range of procedures, the most popular being breast augmentations and liposuction. In 2011 alone nearly 25,000 women had breast enlargements, a further 13,561 had breast reductions and 9,000 more had their breasts lifted to correct sagging. And it wasn't just women: around 8,000 men also had their 'man boobs' surgically reduced. A total of 41,628 people underwent variations of the liposuction procedure which Dr Arolkar had introduced to India around thirty years earlier, while another 15,000 had tummy tucks.

As these figures suggest, plastic surgery in India is huge: 2015 estimates put the worth of its overall cosmetic surgery industry as Rs460 *crore* – around £70 million – which is set to rise to over £17 billion by 2019. As I went up to Dr Arolkar's office I passed publicity posters featuring world-famous Bollywood stars. Styled with an uncharacteristic seriousness, the actors were there to give a well-loved face to the very advanced – and very expensive – surgical offerings of an industry which is now nearly as important to Mumbai as their own.

I was immediately struck by how Dr Arolkar's career had been shaped by a unique combination of clear-sighted ambition, serendipity and an open and creative mind.

'I wanted to do surgery all along, even at university,' the doctor, a slight and kindly man in his sixties, began after apologising for not offering me tea, something that is apparently not allowed in consulting rooms, even if you happen to be a top surgeon. 'In the second year of med school I'd do minor things – biopsies, for example,' he continued. 'Then I started getting interested in scar formation. At that point I met a friend at university – he was from the school of arts – [who] had been developing prostheses through carving and sculpting in silicon rubber.'

Dr Arolkar's admiration for his friend's creations was palpable, and the excitement with which he spoke seemed to dissolve the intervening decades. 'He had made a finger that was so realistic,' he continued, 'it had hairs and pink nails – it looked just like a living finger.' For much of his early career, his medical expertise was put to use for charity and he spent a large part of his free time applying his newfound skills to those disfigured by diseases such as leprosy or severely injured in accidents. In some cases Arolkar had almost miraculous success – a man whose arm was caught in a printing machine and crushed up to the elbow, for example, had the damaged limb's basic function restored and was able to return to work.

The impact made by Dr Arolkar and his team during their periodic and unpaid stints in deprived agricultural and industrial areas was profound, allowing people to return to their communities or support themselves after injuries which a few years before might have been career ending. And they worked hard, completing up to 500 hours of surgery per visit, usually at night. There was often no electricity, no autoclave for sterilising surgical equipment and little to eat. 'We only had boiling water for sterilisation,' he told me, 'and I brought my own tools. When there was a power cut, we would hold a torch up and continue.'

But though the work was gruelling, and undertaken in desperate conditions at a time when cosmetic surgery was still a novelty regarded with some suspicion in India, the hundreds of hours Dr Arolkar and his small band of fellow student doctors put in were valuable in more ways than one.

'In the meantime, I was earning a living as a surgeon in Mumbai,' Arolkar continued. 'Most of my work was to correct hare lips and cleft palates as well as reconstruction following leprosy. At that time, plastic surgery was considered unusual here in the city – you have to be very vain, people said, to do it. It actually took a long time for aesthetic surgery to get into the limelight because it was seen as something unnecessary. So in 1982 nobody really knew what cosmetic surgery was in India.'

This was all set to change, however, and Arolkar's experience would stand him in good stead, as would the 'phenomenal' teaching he received from Dr N. H. Antia, then a leader in plastic surgery who had trained under the famous Sir Harold Gillies. Gillies is known as the 'father of plastic surgery', a visionary surgeon who both pioneered reconstructive surgery techniques on soldiers wounded in the First and Second World Wars and performed some of the first sex-change operations. As attitudes shifted, Arolkar and his small band of specialist colleagues were in prime position.

As Dr Arolkar was talking about the scarcity of plastic surgeons in India even as recently as thirty years ago, I couldn't help thinking how ironic it was that the very first plastic surgeries were performed in ancient India. A form of rhinoplasty is thought to have been invented by an Indian surgeon in around 800 BCE. Though it had already been adopted in a modified form in medieval Italy, the 'Indian nose' came to the attention of British medical professionals and public only during the days of the East India Company. Late in 1794 a curious letter was published in the *Gentleman's Gazette*, a popular London magazine. Signed only 'B.L.', it seems to have been sent from India by an artist, Barak Longmate, who had made an engraving of an Indian cart driver called Cowsajee. Longmate recounts the tale of this former employee of the East India Company who made the error of being captured and imprisoned by Tipu Sultan, the King of Mysore, a region then much coveted by Britain. Already allied with the French East India Company, Tipu

Sultan bore a particular grudge against the British, who had broken a treaty to support his father against the neighbouring Maratha kingdom. With British soldiers and their allies, especially Indian ones, Tipu Sultan was famous for showing no mercy and – even though he had been pensioned by the East India Company after the last Anglo-Indian war had ended two years before – Cowsajee, who unfortunately for him also happened to be Marathi, had his right hand amputated and his nose cut off by Tipu's orders.

Barak Longmate's letter to the *Gentleman's Gazette* recounts how Cowsajee lived without a nose for about a year. He may well have been saving up from his pension during that time because at the end of the twelve months he travelled to Puna to see a surgeon about having a little cosmetic work done on his face. The British doctors who were able to observe the procedure, in which a living graft of skin was cut from the patient's own face to reconstruct the missing nose, were apparently appropriately impressed.

The procedure that Cowsajee underwent – a version of which was still being used by Antia at his Mumbai hospital's Tata Department of Plastic Surgery in the 1980s – would have been developed certainly before 250 BCE and probably around 1500 BCE, when it begins to be obliquely alluded to in ancient texts. It is detailed in the world's oldest written manual on surgery, the *Sushruta Samhita*, which derives from the work of Suśruta, an Ayurvedic physician who may have worked in Varanasi in 1000 or 800 BCE. Suśruta had emphasised surgical training as an integral part of medical education and as the most important part of Ayurveda, an ancient professionalised medical system in India. His *Samhita*, widely thought to have been written down around 600 BCE, painstakingly documented preoperative and postoperative care, diet and surgical indications and contraindications of various diseases such as bowel perforation, hernia, obstetrical injuries, anal fistulae and fractures of the arms and legs. Suśruta developed and applied plastic surgical techniques for reconstructing noses, genitalia and earlobes, among other things, and it is in his work that we first find a description of the 'Indian nose'.

The details of the operation were as follows: a pattern corresponding to the size of the nose to be repaired was cut from the leaf of a creeper. The template was then used to cut a similar shape from the cheek. The cheek skin was sutured with a sharp needle and cotton thread over where the nose would have been. Incisions were made where the nostrils would be and the outer skin was turned in. Two tubes (stalks of the castor oil plant) were inserted into the new nostrils to allow normal breathing and prevent flesh from hanging down. The newly attached cheek flesh was then dusted with three plant-derived powders called Pattanga, Yashtimdhukam and Rasanjana (liquorice, red sandal-wood and barberry) that had been pulverised together. Finally, the nose was enveloped in cotton and several times sprinkled over with pure, refined sesame oil. When the flap of skin removed from the cheek had successfully healed over, any excess skin was removed and tidied up with some final trimming and suturing.

This use of the cheek flap later developed into the similar forehead-flap method that Barak Longmate documented: 'This operation is very generally successful,' he wrote. 'The artificial nose is secure, and looks nearly as well as the natural one; nor is the scar on the forehead very observable after a length of time ... This operation is not uncommon in India and has been practised from time immemorial.'

Unsurprising, then, and perhaps almost inevitable, that thousands of years of experience in aesthetic plastic surgery, a fast-growing cadre of Indian cosmetic surgeons and Bollywood role models willing to embrace the modern Western fashion for self-enhancement should combine to place Mumbaikars at the forefront of India's cosmetic surgery boom.

'The culture changed totally,' Dr Arolkar continued as

we carried on talking over a delicious lunch in the strictly vegetarian hospital canteen. '[Now] people come and say, I want a little tuck here, bigger lips – it's swung like a pendulum the other way. I have been president of the Indian Association of Plastic Surgeons since 2013, though they've now reduced the term to two years because this field has become so popular.' But, as he went on to say, success has brought its own problems for the industry. 'Because of this there are also now a lot of quacks coming up who are not trained in surgery at all ... so insurance premiums and claims are both rising. Regulation is almost absent. We do have a consumer court and a civil court – and technically anyone can go there and complain, but really we need advisory medical bodies and councils to review this.'

Worryingly, an estimated fifty-five per cent of rhinoplasties conducted by reputable Indian plastic surgeons are repairs to those that have gone wrong in the first instance, having been carried out in unregulated, often illegally operated small-town clinics by unqualified practitioners. A 2011 *Times of India* investigation found that patients were often discharged within a few hours of being operated upon. Without regulation, competitive pricing means that, for many patients, the sole determining factor in where they choose to be operated on is cost.

For patients who do pick the wrong surgeon, the consequences can be severe, even fatal. A famous Tollywood (Telugu) actress, Aarthi Agarwal, who was refused liposuction by her Hyderabad surgeon went ahead with the procedure in America. She died, aged thirty-one, of respiratory problems soon after. Aarthi's Indian surgeon had turned her down because she had very little fat under the skin – which is what liposuction is supposed to deal with. The procedure is not appropriate either for removing large amounts of body fat or for treating the 'skinny-fat' phenomenon: the sort of mid-waist fat that is internal, wrapped around the organs, and common in Indians, stemming from either genetics or the pre-natal environment. Add to that the change in many Indians' diets to high-calorie foods, an increasingly sedentary lifestyle and the decline of the perception that big is beautiful and it becomes clear that the demand for liposuction will probably escalate further still.

In the absence of regulation, Dr Arolkar believes the onus has to be on would-be patients to assess their doctor's credentials before going under the knife. 'They also need to be aware of complications,' Dr Arolkar told me. 'But either way the risks of dissatisfaction are high, because now some people don't really know what they want. They say they want to become more beautiful, but they don't know what they want to change! Sometimes I think, actually, you need a brain change, because I've seen people who were asking the impossible.'

I was intrigued that what people are asking for were clearly expensive procedures. In Mumbai, a tummy tuck will set you back more than Rs200,000 – around £2,000. This is ten times cheaper than the United States in absolute terms (though when adjusted for the cost of living the affordability to someone earning an average middle-class Indian salary is probably similar). There'd be a similar price tag on breast augmentation, while a nose job starts at Rs100,000. Why were people willing to spend so much on procedures that, as Dr Arolkar said, would until recently have been seen as entirely unnecessary?

'The thing is, people are becoming more aware of their exterior and showing more of their body, so blemishes get amplified,' Dr Arolkar told me. 'I've had some very strange requests – like one lady asked me to move a mole to another part of her body. Another time, a girl came to me and asked if I could get rid of the smallpox vaccination scar from her upper arm. Then a boy came to me with slightly floppy ears. He was twenty-three. They really weren't all that bad so I told him to go away. He wouldn't, so I asked him for three times as much as it should cost, just to put him off.

He turned up the next day with the money. He had sold the motorbike his father had given him.'

'Do you understand why he was so desperate?' I asked.

'Peer pressure. There was a man from a village in Gujarat who wanted six fingers! Turned out lots of people had that in his village. The thing is, you don't want to look out of the ordinary.' Satish told me how some actresses were asking for breast reductions even in their seventies. 'In the old days, actresses were larger, they had full breasts – in India it was a good thing, it was a sign of fertility.' Traditional representations of the human form in India do seem to have an extensive history of fêting the rotund rather than the svelte. From the rounded stomachs of Harappan adult male and buxom female figurines, to corpulent per- sonifications of scriptural heroes on the shikara of modern temples, beauty has seldom been the ripped abdominals of the classical Greek ideal.

In more recent decades, the perception of the ideal body, at least in Mumbai, has publicly undergone a seismic shift. Instead of looking like the boy next door (with a bit of puppy fat), movie heroes became sexy versions of the incredible hulk. Where actresses were once rounded and buxom, they began to follow a trend towards size zero. Bariatric (stomach stapling) surgeries are big busi- ness (and openly flaunted by politicians, according to Dr Arolkar). Then in 1991 unfavourable economic con- ditions forced devaluation of the rupee and an influx of foreign investment followed. In the ensuing decades the Indian economy almost quadrupled in size. Foreign capital flooded into Bollywood and Bollywood in turn became a global export. Western influence increased with the estab- lishment of MTV and the arrival of international glossy fashion magazines such as *Vogue*. Now, India's fashionable were watching the world – and the world began looking back. Projected onto gigantic screens wherever its diaspora could be found, the exquisite faces and perfect bodies of the

Mumbai film industry's celebrities were constantly before the public gaze – adoring, or critical. It makes perfect sense that Mumbai would embrace cosmetic surgery the way it has. Nowadays, of course, it's not just celebrities who are constantly observed: India also has 118 million active social media accounts. Staying current, including knowing what it means to be beautiful, has never been more immediate.

For those whose jobs require them to stay in the limelight, the pressures are even more acute. In an industry where appearance is everything, there is a particular vulnerability: adoration might turn to career-ending criticism without warning. The media are, of course, only too ready to ridicule anyone who either has surgery or who does not conform to their own version of perfection. It's a lose–lose situation. Unsurprisingly, many celebrities who do have procedures go to great lengths to keep them secret. Dr Arolkar had already cautioned me that talking to an Indian celebrity about their cosmetic surgery would be next to impossible, but I knew of two people who, early on, had broken ranks to speak publicly about plastic surgery: the actress Koena Mitra and one of Bollywood's few female film directors, Farah Khan.

Despite roles in several Bollywood films, Koena's fame as an actress was overshadowed by becoming an exemplar of the perils of plastic surgery. 'She's sort of insignificant now,' a magazine editor told me. 'Her entire career was ruined by bad surgery.' Though I was unable to secure an interview, she has previously commented extensively on her experience, speaking frankly about the choices she had made and the impact they had had on what could have been a significant career in Bollywood.

A former model (with a masters degree in psychology), it's hard to see what could have been improved upon before her surgery in 2011 – after all, that symmetrical face, wide almond eyes and enviable figure had already won her beauty crowns and catwalk gigs. By contrast, in the 'after' photos her face seems more stiff, mask-like. But noticeable though the difference is, the true cost of her nose job was measured in more than aesthetics. Koena said that, after the rhinoplasty, her 'bones started swelling up' and that a series of corrective operations ensued. She was left in severe pain and housebound, while rumours circulated that her face had been so disfigured that it was difficult for her even to smile.

The studios shied away and her career ground to a halt. In a 2014 interview she told the *Times of India*, 'I sat at home initially. But I could not take it any more and started going out with that face of mine … I didn't hide anything. But people spoke and wrote the worst … about me.' She was also quoted in a film magazine talking about the scale of plastic surgery consumerism in Bollywood. 'I can give you a long list of names with their long list of surgeries,' she said. 'My list of surgeries is really tiny compared to many leading stars of the day. I at least had the courage to come out and talk.' And though her face has recovered, it is no longer one that mainstream Bollywood has since deemed attractive enough to cast.

Farah Khan, by contrast, has become a hero to some after owning up to post-pregnancy surgery of the sort Dr Arolkar says is increasingly popular: the 'mommy-make-over'. Khan started as a choreographer before becoming one of Bollywood's biggest producer-directors (with block-buster credits including *Om Shanti Om*). Though she has appeared on screen, Farah is not the type to be seen in hot pants or tiny sari blouses, as Bollywood's impossibly lithe starlets tend to. Rather, her figure is more like the average woman's. Usually undertaken by women who want no more children, the 'mommy-makeover' comprises one or more procedures designed to counter the effects of preg-nancy and active motherhood.

A few years after giving birth to triplets, and after researching the procedure thoroughly, she decided the hanging tummy she was left with and which dieting and exercise had failed to budge would have to go. When I spoke to her, her openness about double standards and women reclaiming their bodies after having children was refreshing. One of the 'problems' of being a celebrity is the back catalogue of available photographs that provide the media with ready-made 'before' and 'after' comparisons.

Women do come under far closer scrutiny in this respect than men. Even when some of Bollywood's favourite male actors fall prey, they usually get off with the odd mentions of wrinkles filled. In India, as everywhere else, women's bodies are perceived as fair game, hotness before childbirth mutating into mummy yumminess after. But, as Farah has often stated, 'There is nothing to hide.'

Celebrities who stand up for themselves post-surgery in the press or social media are still relatively rare, but they do exist. Actress Anushka Sharma spoke out recently 'to end the noise', as she put it, after a barrage of tweets criticising her newly augmented lips. 'I felt bullied. I didn't know that people could be so mean,' she told the newspapers. 'Some of the stuff was quite funny but some of it was such pure vitriol that I cried. It's because we don't reply to them that people think they can get away with anything. I didn't think I had to inform the world before getting my lips enhanced. It's my body and my decision.' In 2015, Shilpa Shetty (actress and star of Celebrity Big Brother in the UK) also admitted to having had four nose jobs; and the legendary Zeenat Aman came out publicly in support of cosmetic surgery in general. 'To each his own … I'm in favour of it,' she said.

Where Bollywood stars go, everyone else follows, from the older generations to what Dr Arolkar calls 'nubile teenagers' who want 'dream' bodies. But it's no longer just about the more complex surgeries allowing women (and men) to emerge with better breasts or smaller waistlines. The cultural change Dr Arolkar had described to me had also, in recent years, extended to an explosion in what he called 'office-procedures' – faster, easier, cheaper and less risky quick fixes that take minutes instead of hours.

'Once you look good, you only want to look better. Human nature! If something is available and affordable the beneficiary of a previous cosmetic procedure hankers for more. So people are opting more and more for these – like lasers for quick fixes, Botox and fillers.'

The first dermal filler approved for cosmetic use was collagen derived from cows. That was in the USA in 1981, since which time dozens of laboratory-made injectable filling agents have been developed. Botox was first used in Canada in 1992 and the big boom in 'office procedures' started building in India around a decade later. Today, with China, India has the fastest-growing market in Asia for such off-the-shelf cosmetic work.

I decided to meet a doctor who had filled, layered smoothed and sculpted Mumbai's elite without ever lifting a scalpel. As my taxi pulled up outside her Bandra apartment on a pretty, tree-lined street, Dr Rashmi Shetty waved to my daughter and me, guiding us up from her second-floor balcony. Around forty, with clear skin, lustrous black hair and a conventional Indian beauty, she could easily be mistaken for an actress or model herself, an image which must also have been an excellent advertisement for her own practice.

Though she had been an accomplished dancer, Rashmi's real talent was in medicine. I had been corresponding with her by email, trying to find a time when she wouldn't be studying for further professional qualifications, writing articles for medical journals or lecturing at national or international conferences and seminars. We'd managed to find a slot and met over breakfast. Disarmingly friendly and whip-smart, she made the interview feel more like a relaxed conversation with a good friend than a rushed session with a woman who had everyone who was anyone in Bollywood knocking at her clinic door.

'I always wanted to be a surgeon,' Dr Shetty began as we, and our daughters tucked into aloo parathas and chai. 'I got into general surgery and my initial postings were in plastic surgery – that's where I started liking tissue reconstruction, realising how we can put a face back together in a beautiful way. I realised how important looks were to people. To a patient, that small mark on a face could be a reminder of abuse, or a burning, or a disease. For many people beauty is not just vanity. The way you look can change your whole life course.'

As Rashmi recounted stories from her surgical training and of her voluntary work for Smile Train – a charity providing corrective surgery for children with cleft lips and palates – she also alluded to the rapidly growing appetite of Mumbaikars for cosmetic surgery. Fourteen years earlier, when she stopped working as a surgeon proper and first set up as an 'aesthetic physician', 'I sat there for six hours a day and not a patient turned up. So gradually I went down to two hours a day on alternate days,' she said. 'A few years later patients started spilling over. I never advertise, I don't even have a board outside my clinic. Now, I see up to sixteen patients a day. A consultation takes twenty minutes and the treatments, if they decide to have one, take twenty minutes to an hour.'

Rashmi's clientele includes some of Bollywood's biggest names, male and female, and they have not been shy in praising what 'Bollywood's favourite aesthetic physician' has been able to do for them. On the ratings-topping chat show *Koffee with Karan*, Rakhi Sawant, a Mumbai celebrity best known simply for being famous, declared, 'My doctor is Rashmi Shetty … as they say, what God didn't give, the doctor gives instead.' 'But that was at the time I did her face,' Rashmi clarified, laughing. 'Now she has had other procedures done – *not* my work.'

Even those willing to admit to cosmetic procedures seem reluctant to go into detail. Shilpa Shetty (no relation), wrote about how she trusted Rashmi's knowledge of skin; Sania Mirza, a world number one women's doubles tennis player, praised her for producing results that other doctors couldn't; and Anita Dongre, one of India's best known fashion designers added, 'What kept me from going to aesthetic doctors was my apprehension for anything invasive and drastic. [Rashmi] just fixed me with the least that there can be.' There are many, many endorsements in this vein, but needles don't get a single mention.

Such vagueness is perhaps intended to maintain a myth of beauty naturally enhanced, rather than medically manipulated. Ethically, of course, Rashmi could disclose no individual details, but her website makes clear the procedures on offer, ranging from simple skin treatments such as laser and retexturing to fillers that would pump up lips, sculpt facial features and iron out wrinkles, plus, naturally, Botox and treatments for baldness.

I visited her clinic in nearby Santa Cruz, where Rashmi told me about the 'vampire facelift' – a bizarre procedure familiar to some from the 'after' shots of their blood-smeared faces posted online by both Kim Kardashian and Israeli model Bar Refaeli. The procedure uses the patient's own blood, separating out the fraction containing the platelets, growth factors and stem cells and then injecting what's left into multiple sites on the face. The initial result is a gruesome mess, but it remains a favourite of celebrities in the West, allegedly helping the body to repair itself, rebuilding collagen and thus rejuvenating the skin. I couldn't imagine any of Rashmi's Mumbai celebrity clients showing off their bloodied and swollen faces so freely; that would hardly fit the immaculate image most Bollywood actors project, even if the procedure is helping them maintain it.

As it turned eleven a.m. the influx of clients began, and while Rashmi juggled consultations and preparation for medical procedures with perfect ease, I sat in her waiting room and watched the passing show. As I leafed through the coffee table magazines in the waiting room, admiring yachts, poring over the articles in *Millionaire Asia*, dermatology journals and women's magazines, a receptionist offered me a patient form to fill in. 'Oh, I'm just here to interview Rashmi,' I explained, as she apologised and took the paperwork away. I can't say it wasn't tempting: at thirty-nine, I was probably already nearly two decades older than some of her clients and after looking at images of what filling, sculpting, lifting and plumping could do I had started to see things wrong with my face that I hadn't noticed before.

Perhaps it was due to watching those droves of people come and go as if they were simply visiting a dentist or a hairdresser, that the whole thing was starting to appear completely normal. I took a moment to post a status update on Facebook about how easy it would be to have some filler. If there had been a 'dislike' button, it would have saved my friends the time they took to write lengthy comments asking whether I'd gone mad and pleading with me not to do it.

My temptation (which I conquered) clearly wasn't an isolated one – I had first come across Rashmi while reading an article in the *Times of India* headlined 'Mumbai's got a serial cosmetic surgery club'. As the headline suggests, it reported how the quest for the Bollywood ideal of bodily perfection had become all-consuming, both inside and outside the industry. I had noticed that many of Rashmi's clients were middle-aged women, presumably in search of rejuvenation. Surely, though, there must be a downside?

'People understand the risk, yes, they do, but they say let's go ahead and do it,' Rashmi told me. 'The next woman from the party has become thinner, let's do it. Thin is very desirable – to the extent that women try to get into their teenage daughters' clothes – but older women need a fat percentage: your overall weight distribution changes with age. But they all want to maintain a waistline. We are fighting the natural [ageing process] – they cut down on carbs so much they come to me with hair falling out, with dark circles under their eyes ...'

I could see how it could easily become a vicious circle and how quick-fix procedures would become desirable, even necessary, to people whose lives were not lived in front of audiences of hundreds of millions.

'My patients are mostly from the film industry, but there are also bank employees, teachers, housewives – today everyone wants to look beautiful. I have lots of male patients now too. Before, if there was one scratch to their car men would get annoyed, yet they didn't seem to care about how they themselves looked,' Rashmi joked.

Indeed, though I didn't see any men in Rashmi's waiting room while I was there, most of my companions were just ordinary citizens – an older woman, probably in her late fifties, wearing a bindi on her forehead and a traditional salwar kameez; another woman in her late twenties maybe, in jeans; another in her early thirties wearing a mini skirt; and a fourth girl in ripped jeans and comfortable loafers.

While I waited, I chatted with a woman in her twenties who had moved to Mumbai from Tanzania to go to medical school. 'I think in this period in time we are very self-conscious,' she told me. 'Even as a doctor, when a patient comes to you, they look up to you and if I have pimple, they think, why doesn't she take care of herself? Or if we tell them to lose weight, then we have to be fit too. Even my mother is a patient here. She has Botox. She was sceptical the first time, so Rashmi did half her face to show her how it would compare. Rashmi does not want her to look unnatural – she says you should age gracefully. And every year my mother comes from Tanzania to see her.'

One of the more interesting improvements Rashmi offered was skin lightening. Cosmetic skin-lightening products are a sizeable industry in India, with 'before and after' advertisements on billboards across the country and pages of classified bridal ads in the *Times of India* every Sunday seeking 'Slim, Fair, B'ful girl'; 'beautiful, professionally qualified, fair Hindu girl'; 'seeking cultured fair beautiful girl'; 'Qualified, Fair, Slim girl'; 'Beautiful tall girl for very fair, handsome vegetarian boy' …

'The ideal of beauty is light skin,' Rashmi explained to me. 'Actually you can look like a frog. But the ideal bride is a woman with light skin; at front desks in offices the receptionist should have light skin. We are not one "race" in India – we have so called Aryan, Mongolian, Dravidian types. So we are used to working with different skin. Even in south India, where people are thought of as darker-skinned, the Iyengars [high caste Brahmans] are lighter; in Mangalore people are lighter. I used to think the desire to be lighter was socio-economic but now I don't – we don't get lower economic groups at our practice. But the thing is, if you are dark, it is harder to maintain an even skin tone, so I think it's more about that than a particular shade. The biggest thing people come to me for is skin tone or colour. But tone can change with facial structure. For example, the area below the eye can get sunken with age and that can give the appearance of dark circles. So changes on the skin cannot be addressed by changing the actual skin tone alone – I have to also look at the tissue and face structure. You need to work beyond the skin with all the layers to get an even skin tone.'

Though that was what Rashmi's clients came to her to address, in India there is undeniably a very deeply rooted worship of light skin colour, as the matrimonials illustrate. I remember an English friend of mine being taken aback when I told him that Bollywood actors were actually Indian. 'But they're all so white,' he said. 'Are you sure?' Today, of course, they're not all Indian. A few have one south Asian and one white parent; many films have formulaic nightclub scenes with backing dancers who are entirely European – and generally also all blonde.

In terms of ideals of beauty, in India people with light skin and/or eyes occupy a place of privilege for a variety of perceived reasons: dark skin is associated with poverty because the poor are more likely to work in the harsh sun; it may also be associated with underprivileged classes or castes. Blame is variously laid with the Persians, Aryans, or the British, or Westernisation. They point to the traditionally dark skin colour of certain Hindu gods; the description in ancient epics of dark-skinned princesses celebrated as great beauties in a time before white was right.

The reality, as Rashmi had alluded to, is that outward appearance and status in a country as populous as India is far more nuanced by geography and genetics. A friend of mine, a doctor from a so-called low 'untouchable' caste, is not dark skinned at all (and has green eyes). My mother's family consists of nine siblings and close relatives who vary from having extremely dark skin to almost white. Among them they also have a pick and mix of dark brown, hazel, green and blue eyes. None the less, however flawed the reasons that link whiteness with desirability might be, the fact is that it still exists.

There are those who hope to bring down this chromatocracy and several activist movements (whose membership lists include some Bollywood stars) have united against the products and advertisers, while the non-Bollywood film industry produces many thoughtful films employing more natural-looking actors. There is also the 'Dark is Beautiful' campaign, launched in 2013 by actress and producer Nandita Das, which aims to promote the celebration of 'beauty beyond colour'.

It could be a losing battle. A 2012 BBC news story reported more sales of skin-lightening creams in India than Coca-Cola and featured a shower gel that claimed to whiten the genitals of Indian women. It was promoted with a television advert showing a (fair-skinned) wife, first ignored by her handsome husband and then ecstatically reunited with him after using the product. The skin-whitening industry is now worth an estimated £283 million. Even-handedly, it doesn't exclude those without vaginas: like the 'Fair & Lovely' skin-lightening cream marketed to women, 'Fair & Handsome' has hired heavyweight brand ambassadors in the form of Bollywood megastars Shah Rukh Khan and Hrithik Roshan. Nor does the marketing stop with 'fairness' products. There is an amusing, often politically-incorrect range of tonics, potions and even exercise equipment that reek of quackery, targeted at the uncritical. I'd even seen an ad campaign for a product promising to 'increase your height or your money back', pasted on the backs of auto-rickshaws. The watchdogs are reacting. In 2015 the Food and Drug Administration issued notices for, and physically seized two steroid-containing fairness creams: UB Fair for men and No Scars cream for women. The products contained steroids like fluocinolon acetonid and mometasone as well as skin bleaching agents, the side effects of which include skin thinning, rashes, and even excess facial hair growth over time.

Knowing the risks, and thinking of those ubiquitous and miraculous billboard transformations I had seen, I was curious to hear from Rashmi why so many people persist in using them, and whether these creams really work.

'Yes, they do. Companies have a responsibility to stand behind their claims, but the extent of change customers get can be very, very small. Usually, creams include some form of sunscreen. Plant extracts such as liquorice, mulberry or any of the acids that block enzymes of the melanin pathway. Also hydroquinone, which actually bleaches the skin, or light reflective particles. Product engineering has improved so much now that you get that instant satisfaction. There are gold and glitter particles to make skin look like it's glowing. And then people get to like the glow so they keep using it.'

Hydroquinone is recommended for the gradual bleaching of areas of hyper-pigmented skin – spots of uneven skin tone, for example – although many, even most, users of the product apply it to their whole face. The effect is not permanent and, though the compound is approved for human use, laboratory and animal tests indicate that possible side effects may include some cancers or DNA modification.

Many of the women of typically marriageable age in Rashmi's clinic did seem to be there for various skin issues, though at least they were consulting a professional rather than taking the DIY route.

Occasionally, well-off teenagers will ask Rashmi to carry out even more invasive procedures.

'I tell them to go away,' she said. 'Here, even kids have access to money. The parents give it and no one asks them how they spend it. It's like maybe how we went to a hairdressers or a beauty salon, they go to the cosmetic surgeon. They haven't finished growing yet and their faces are going to change. They ask for very specific things some of them, sixteen-year-olds wanting certain parts of their faces sculpted or filled. "Make it thinner here, put in fillers there." I ask them why and they say, "Because I don't like my face at that angle. It doesn't look good in selfies."'

When I thought about it, it made a lot of sense that teens were feeling an increased pressure to go to extremes in the name of appearance. Like the rest of the world, Indian teenagers post 'fat-shaming' photos on Facebook and some young victims have been driven to suicide. For the selfie generation, everyone is in the limelight.

As I left Rashmi to her continuing influx of patients the very beautiful, Brooklyn-born, half-Czech Bollywood actress Nargis Fakhri was due through the door. Seeing her on the Cannes red carpet a few weeks later, statuesque, with her characteristic filler-plumped lips, brought to mind her endorsement of Rashmi's book *Age Erase*: 'There's always extra pressure when it comes to being in the limelight. Not to mention just being a woman who will inevitably go through life's processes. We all want to look and feel young ...' In an interview on the web, she made her reflections on cosmetic surgery even clearer. 'Things fall, gravity happens,' she said. 'You kind of need an extra something as you get older ... so listen, I think technology is great, you know ... I think it's nice to have that option. And I think, why should we not look as hot as a twenty-five-year-old when we are forty-five.'

Rashmi Shetty and Satish Arolkar's Mumbai patients would surely have agreed, but such ideas have their critics too. In the words of one protester in Bangalore, 'If a woman is judged only by the size of her breasts and her hips, then it is shameful not just to Indian women, but to women all over the world.' But if the projections for the unrelenting rise of the most commercialised area of Indian medicine hold true, then there is no turning back now.

In the meantime, across India's great cities, a phenomenon even newer than cosmetic surgery is also gaining pace: the rapid rise of smartly outfitted gym franchises that provide a slower, tougher but healthier route to making the body changes we now crave. Although India's largest gym chain started (in Mumbai) as long ago as 1932, within the last 5 years Talwalkars has more than doubled the number of its offerings, now with 146 'ultramodern branches' across 80 Indian cities. Toward this expansion into India's new urban demographics, in 2012, it partnered with Britain's David Lloyd Leisure Group, with whom they consulted on providing leisure and sports clubs in high-end residential developments, gated community townships and corporate campuses. Fitness First launched in 2008, followed by Gold's Gym and other independent five-star offerings that included women's-only areas or sessions and the type of yoga classes restyled for the West and reintroduced to the new world of fitness in India alongside new staples such as Pilates and Zumba. Even today the concept still has a beautiful novelty. Talwalkars alone now has in excess of 125,000 members who contribute to the company's 28 million USD revenues, but there is much more growth to come: as a nascent fitness market, only around 0.05 per cent of urban Indians have a health club membership, compared to 3.11 per cent in the Asia-Pacific region, 13.2 per cent in Britain, and 17.5 per cent in the USA.

WITH INCREASING INTEREST in looking good by getting fit, wearable tech is also beginning to explode: in 2015, more than 72 million wearable devices were shipped to India, with FitBit, Samsung, Xiaomi and Apple products leading the way. Reports are that Indian manufacturers are not far behind: Micromax-owned YU Televentures, makers of mobile phones and related tech, for example, is betting on its health tracker, YuFit for future growth. As the company's tag line and web address, *Yuplaygod* seems a resonant echo of Bollywood celebrity Rakhi Sawant's rationale for using medical technology to improve the things god didn't quite get right.

Via the scalpel, elliptical trainer or app, as the pressures on Mumbaikars to become and stay beautiful remain enormous, the quest for physical perfection in India's wealthiest city has never been so popular, or so accessible.

3

Knowledge for Long Life

SOUTH OF MUMBAI, the skyscrapers of the city are soon replaced by verdant mountains and then lithe coconut palms which frame the sea and envelop the land. As the Konkan route exits Maharashtra, it runs past the modest homes, churches, mosques and forests of three more states – Goa, Karnataka and finally, Kerala. The two-day drive is undeniably beautiful and opens a window onto an India very different from the traffic-clogged, unrelenting urban sprawl of Mumbai. Much like the rich blue of the sky, shades of green on the ground are a welcome respite to the eye and a delight to the lungs. The Ghat mountain range that flanks India's western coast ranks seventh in the world's biodiversity hotspots, and along it the variety of plant life flourishing in this part of India becomes apparent. Among the prolific coconut palms are mango trees and cashews; Flame of the Forest trees crowned with mushroom clouds of crimson; emerald expanses of rice paddies; grand jackfruit trees, heavy with enormous, reptilian-skinned dark green fruit and with their trunks masked entirely by black pepper vines.

Such plants have been used in Indian medical traditions for thousands of years, and in particular by Ayurveda. I was making the journey to discover more about the use of herbs in one of India's oldest native medical practices – and how the ancient discipline was faring against mainstream medicine. I knew that Western doctors had been studying and working with Ayurveda much longer than many suppose: in fact, the trade in the precious 'black gold' from the pepper vines and other medicinal spices I had seen was one of the great draws for fifteenth-century Europeans seeking out medicines, as well as exotic flavours. The lure of these valuable substances would also bring them into contact with a natural world largely unknown and mysterious, as well as diseases such as cholera and dysentery that they had never encountered before.

The medicine practised in Europe at the time was based on a very different system from that of today. Medical knowledge in Europe during the Early Modern period was based on the 2,000-year-old tradition influenced by the writings of Hippocrates, Aristotle, Galen and Avicenna. According to their classical medical theories, it was imbalances in the four humours – blood (hot and wet), phlegm (cold and wet), black bile (cold and dry), yellow bile (hot and dry) – that were the cause of fevers and disease, and they were remedied through diet, purges, bleeding and plant- and mineral-derived remedies. The concept of balance restoring health and imbalance undermining it would have been familiar in Asia and one upon which much of India's folk and scholarly medical theory was also based. Many of these ideas were recorded in core Indian medical texts like the *Sushruta* and *Charaka Samhitas* dating between the ninth and sixth centuries BCE (and lost books it refers to, like the *Atreya*, and *Agnivesa* treatises). But they were also rooted in key 'books' of the Hindu scriptures – the *Rigveda* and *Atharvaveda* – which preceded these medical texts by around a thousand years.

On 12 March 1534 a young doctor from a Portuguese Jewish family boarded a ship at Lisbon, bound for the west coast of India. It is likely that Garcia de Orta, who had been forcibly converted to Christianity under the reign of terror of the Spanish Inquisition, chose to escape persecution by taking a job 4,500 nautical miles away, as attendant physician to his military patron, Martim Afonso de Sousa, who had also commanded the first official Portuguese expedition to Brazil. De Orta served de Sousa during campaigns from the Kathiawar peninsula north of Mumbai, along the Arabian Sea to the south-eastern tip of India and into Sri Lanka.

From the age of fifteen until he left Iberia at thirty-four, Garcia de Orta had studied and then lectured in medicine and natural and moral philosophy. As his captain general's military campaigns ended, he settled in Goa and set up a lucrative medical practice that he would oversee until his death thirty years later. As well as working as a doctor, de Orta dedicated himself to recording the use of more than eighty drugs, fruits, spices, minerals and medicinal preparations either found in India or employed there. He was clearly fascinated by the ancient and sophisticated medicines he had found in the subcontinent, planting botanical gardens both at his home in Goa and on his estate in Mumbai – very close to where the British-built Mumbai town hall stands today. He had agents – shopkeepers, traders, soldiers, translators, travellers, missionaries – send him plants and seeds from around India and he gathered information from discussions with Indian physicians, slaves, servant boys, cooks and gardeners. The information he collected was published in 1563 as *Colloquies on the Simples and Drugs of India* and it provided the Western and Eastern worlds with an early opportunity to explore the interaction both between old and new forms of knowledge and between Indian and European medical systems.

In India, both Portuguese migrants and Indian aristocracy came to de Orta suffering from conditions he would never have encountered in his own country. Undaunted, he adapted to his new practice: using taste and smell, he deduced what balancing properties – cold, hot, dry or wet – his new collections of herbs, seeds and drugs might have and prescribed accordingly. He experimented both on his patients and on himself, turning to Indian medical practices when his European methods failed and making their medicinal herbs famous among Westerners in India as well as back in Europe. By the time Goa's Royal Hospital opened in the sixteenth century, both Indian physicians and folk healers were working alongside European doctors. The hybrid medical knowledge established there was enormously successful, and being adopted by the Portuguese seaborne empire, had spread to the hospitals of Lisbon and Coimbra by the eighteenth century.

I first came across de Orta through an exhibition hosted by the National Centre for Biological Sciences in Bangalore, which examined botanical interaction between the East and West during the pre-colonial period. Among botanical illustrations, prints and maps was the *Hortus Indicus Malabaricus*, a study of the medicinal plants of the Malabar (a region beginning in south Goa and encompassing Kerala) between 1678 and 1703. Commissioned by Hendrik van Rheede, an aristocrat who had been governor of Dutch Malabar, it was an ordered catalogue of nearly 800 paintings. Van Rheede had left home aged fourteen to join the Dutch East India Company and had developed there a strong and mutually respectful relationship with Indian scholars and physicians, three of whom became contributors to his text. He also worked with Itty Achudem, traditional physician from the lower-castes who was an expert on local plants used in medicinal and culinary formulations, and whose medical palm leaf manuscript is thought to have been handed down through his family to the present day.

Curious to learn more about the pre-British colonial history of Indian medicines, I spoke to the curator of the exhibition, Dr Annamma Spudich, a scientist formerly of Stanford University who was born and raised in Kerala. I was fascinated by how – and why – a geneticist who had built her career firmly within the American university system had switched to the study of Indian scientific traditions. We chatted about the long trips she takes several times a year to Europe, Bangalore and Kerala, where she has been recording the work of India's few remaining Ashtavaidyas, practitioners of a specialist branch of India's Ayurvedic medicine.

The Ashtavaidya's tradition had arisen from a historic interaction between text-based Ayurveda practices and regional folk medicine that drew on Kerala's medicinal flora. Roughly translating from the Sanskrit as 'the science of longevity', Ayurveda is based on a theory of medicine originating in Brahmanic tradition and set down in Sanskrit texts in the early centuries of the Christian era. Its medical theory is based on humoral, physiological and pathological principles of a body in health and disease. Ayurveda covers an enormous number of practices and philosophy, from physical exercise and meditation (yoga) to diet, but at its heart it revolves around the three concepts of *dosha*, *dhātu* and *mala*. *Dhātu* are the body's tissues and *mala* are its waste products. *Dosha* is a little more tricky to capture, but it is often equated with Hippocrates' humours – though in Ayurveda there are three, not four. The *doshas* are semi-fluid substances in the body which regulate its state of balance. Of them, *pitta* and *kapha* seem to align with bile and phlegm, while the third, known as *vāta*, represents wind. The *doshas* interact with the body's waste products and what are referred to as its seven constituents, namely blood, chyle (a milky fluid of lymph and emulsified fats), flesh, fat, bone, marrow and semen. Balance through moderation in all things is the way of Ayurveda – followers of the system are recommended only ever to take reasonable quantities of food, medicines, sleep, sex and exercise, so that the central process of the body, digestion, can do its work, allowing *ojas*, energy, to be extracted.

In general, the medicines used in Ayurveda have plant

and animal origins. In some formulations, minerals and metals, including sulphur, arsenic, lead, copper and gold, have a central role, an innovation that was introduced around CE 1000. Around the same time, opium (historically prescribed for diarrhoea) began to be adopted, it is thought from Islamic sources. As this suggests, India's most ancient living medicine has continually experimented, evolved and absorbed elements from other systems of treatment. Neither has it been uncritical of itself – Ayurveda today has been shaped by revisions and criticisms from within as well as from outside sources. As early as 1698 a *vaidya* (Ayurvedic doctor) by the name of Vīreśvara published a text debating illness and health in which he questioned the whole theory of humoral balance of *doshas*, adding for good measure, 'it resembles the babbling of lunatics'.

I asked Anna about the idea that the study and veneration of plants were part of the culture of India. 'Absolutely,' she said. 'I grew up in Kerala. On my mother's side we had many friends who were traditional physicians, vaidyas. We would call the vaidya as often as we went to the medical doctor. The vaidyas might prescribe a *thailum*, an oil, or maybe the extracts of two or three plants. We'd go to them for a large number of ailments. Of course, if you had appendicitis you'd go to the medical doctor, but from the vaidya we learned about plants that could help us. But this is how we learnt about plants – for an upset stomach, say, my grandmother would tell us to go to the garden and pick these leaves.'

I KNEW THAT, for minor ailments, my mother's family in Tamil Nadu also called this *pattivaidyam* (granny doctor) or *veetuvaidyam* (home doctor). In their part of India this involved a mix of a system known as *Siddha* medicine. This is a system similar to Ayurveda in theory of causes of disease but different in origin; in the types of medicines used and in the ways they are processed; and with its own texts written mainly in Tamil, not Sanskrit. As well as Siddha, there were folk medicines handed down the generations and prescribed by mothers, grannies and relatives within the home – often simply from the spice cupboard in the kitchen. Like the Ashtavaidyas' practice of Ayurveda, these home remedies were the result of an interaction between Indian medical theory and folk knowledge.

'THAT'S ALSO PART of the folklore of medicine', Anna said. 'Indian food is medicine. There is that overlap between them, inbuilt into the cuisine. There have always been these medical traditions, botanical-medical knowledge, massage therapy and so on. I was delivered by a local midwife, and for all of the problems that arose these women knew what medicine to administer. All this was part of our traditional systems – a new mother was bathed for thirty days with extract of certain leaves and roots, some of which helped with the contraction of the uterus – these women had a list of procedures and medicines of their own.

'It wasn't until I was a teenager that a medical college was opened in Kerala. Now there are many medical schools and biomedicine is the dominant system. People want immediate relief with a single-molecule drug rather than wait for the lower concentrations found in traditional medicines to work.' Anna's point was a significant one. Despite the fact that, according to the World Health Organisation, seventy per cent of people in India still use traditional medical therapy as a first line of defence, the way of thinking about medicine and the time frame in which results are expected have changed significantly. We want quick fixes rather than the protracted lifestyle changes that Ayurveda prescribes.

'You should come to Kerala with me and see how the physicians practise. There is a young Ashtavaidya who is trying very hard to preserve the traditions. He's studying at an Ayurveda college. There is not much of the real tradition left.' Anna knew better than most how threatened the history of Ayurveda had become. She'd been devastated to discover that the palm-leaf manuscript that Achudem spoke of in the *Malabaricus* had recently been thrown away by his family. 'It seems to have been suspended in the main house in a hanging basket and they weren't sure what it was, so they put it in the rubbish. It was very sad,' she said, clearly frustrated. Perhaps even more sad is the fact that the loss of Achudem's treasure is by no means an isolated case.

What Anna was saying reminded me of something van Rheede had written in the *Hortus Malabaricus*: that, even in 1678, the use of Indian plants 'whose curative virtues were proclaimed by indigenous physicians as having been famous for extreme antiquity was rapidly approaching its end'.

A further reason for the demise of the Ashtavaidya's work – which would have been a problem even when van Rheede was searching for collaborators in seventeenth-century India – had also emerged from Anna's research. The traditional education of the old Indian medical scholar-practitioners was exclusive, sometimes dependent on royal patronage and extremely long and demanding. Generally, such instruction was given only to men who were members of an existing practitioner's family or of a high caste. A wealthy sponsor would also be vital in order to support what could be fifteen years of rigorous one-to-one apprenticeship. Students would receive training in not only healing practices (study of the medical texts, diagnosis and preparation or medicine formulations) but also logic, astrology and additional periods of meditation and memorisation and recitation of classical texts.

This unwieldy system persisted until the nineteenth century, when a European-style fixed curriculum was introduced, with specialist subject teachers, a set training period and qualifying exams. Successful candidates would receive a medical certificate and a licence permitting practice. Ayurvedic and other traditional medical colleges in India still operate with a standardised syllabus that includes Western disciplines – anatomy, physiology, biochemistry – ostensibly so that the old and new can interact with ease. Although this streamlined system has turned out large numbers of traditional medical physicians and widened the availability of their services, the inclusion of Western practices is considered by many to have undermined the philosophy behind Ayurvedic medicine.

Still, things have been worse. In 1822 the British Raj outlawed the integrative approach pioneered by de Orta and colonial India's various fledgling medical institutions would teach only the separate disciplines, rather than pushing for the pluralism which had been so effective.

Unsurprisingly, under the British, European medicine was to supplant all others. The English politician Thomas Babington Macaulay was the architect of this change. An uncompromising modernist and the son of a missionary, he considered the 'pagan' Indian systems of medicine to be both backward and slowing the progress of Anglicisation. Despite the protests of British Orientalists, he decreed that Ayurveda as a system of medicine was to end. At the new Calcutta Medical College, only one system was to be taught as medicine.

IT IS UNDERSTOOD that much of Vedic medical anatomical knowledge arose as a result of animal sacrifice, rather than opening the human body. Far pre-dating that, such information was gathered from hunting and butchering. India's 20,000-year-old Mesolithic art repeatedly portrays so called 'X-ray' animal images on the walls of rock shelters: complex drawings of boar and cattle showing organs in place. Later came the substantive surgical works of Sushruta, whose texts include a systematic method for the dissection of the human cadaver. But by the nineteenth century, human dissection was not performed as part of the training of Ayurvedic doctors.

ALTHOUGH THERE WERE ARABIC translations of the *Sush-ruta Samhita*, made in the eighth century, the work was not readable in English until 1907. Macaulay read neither Arabic, nor Sanskrit. This must have contributed to his con-clusions as outlined in his 'minute on education', where he described India's offerings as including 'medical doctrines which would disgrace an English farrier, astronomy which would move laughter in girls at an English boarding school …' And so, in 1836, Macaulay famously ordered a fifty-gun salute at the new College to celebrate what was publicised as the first post-mortem dissection of a human body per-formed by an Indian. Despite the circus, and political and practical challenges, practitioners of Ayurveda and other Indian medical systems didn't give up the fight. Encour-aged by the growing strength of nationalist voices towards the 1940s, and in response to the hostility of the colonial policy toward Indian medicine, traditional therapists joined forces and specialised colleges of 'indigenous medicine' were established.

I had a very personal interest in wanting to understand the story of Indian medicine because of my grandfather's involvement in both Ayurveda and post-independence health policy, and an academic one in wishing to under-stand whether Ayurvedic theory and modern science could really be happy bedfellows. After nearly seventy years of independence, and twenty years after the establishment of the government department for Indian systems of medicine for which my grandfather had striven, I was keen to find out where the long struggle between autonomy and integration stood in the twenty-first century.

I arranged to meet an old friend in Bangalore who had trained as an Ayurvedic doctor at a college affiliated to the medical university of Chennai. Anusha had grown up in a house obliquely opposite mine in the Caribbean, before moving to the States in the late 1980s and then to India. There she became fluent in Hindi and learnt Tamil and scholarly Sanskrit so that she could work with ancient Ayurvedic texts. On returning to the States she'd researched complementary and integrative medical therapies with colleagues at Boston University School of Medicine and at the Harvard School of Public Health, which had pointed her towards her main area of interest: Ayurvedic research and development.

Before we met in India, Anusha mentioned that she had been working as a consultant for L'Oréal India in Bangalore. I was curious about what a French cosmetics company would be doing with Indian medicinal herbs. I discovered that, in April 2013, it had opened a research facility in Bangalore's fashionable Whitefield neighbourhood, attracted by the city's reputation for bioinformatics (analysing and storing biological data) and phytochemistry (chemical analysis of the substances derived from plants). In the words of Laurent Attal, the company's executive vice-president of research and innovation, 'This Research and Innovation centre is a tribute to India's scientific excellence. It is designed to become a laboratory of innovation for Indian beauty and a source of inspiration for the rest of the world.'

L'Oréal India's initial bridge products between traditional beauty routines and modern technology had included rudimentary fusions with familiar Indian beauty regimes – Garnier Shampoo plus Oil; Maybelline Colossal Kajal – but their interest in working with Ayurvedic specialists was part of a three-year investment programme costing approximately £110 million, designed to uncover the secrets of plants used in Ayurveda that might turn up leads to improved cosmetics. It looked like L'Oréal was working on a hunch that the next anti-ageing revelation might well be found in the ancient herbs used by Ayurvedic healers.

L'Oréal aside, Anusha's academic interest was in the medicinal rather than cosmetic, researching the safety and efficacy of traditional Ayurvedic formulations. In fact, they are on the world's radar just as much as Indianised mascara and maquillage. The market for Ayurvedic products has been growing steadily at ten to twelve per cent annually and now boasts a Rs8–10,000 *crore* (£8–10 million) turnover combining both domestic and exports. In addition, although it is difficult to put an exact figure on what proportion of the medical tourism industry (worth about £2.5 billion) is attributable to Ayurveda, there are signs that it is significant, probably particularly in Kerala, where traditional Ayurvedic spas have long been a major attraction for foreign tourists.

Though her clear commitment to Ayurveda, its holistic philosophy and its efficacy was understandable, much of Anusha's recent work had involved investigation of concerns regarding the safety of traditional medicines that had been surfacing in medical literature from several countries, particularly Italy and the USA. In the United States and in Europe, herbal products don't necessarily have to be classified as medicines: they can be marketed as cosmetic or food products. This means that, in general, consumers regard them as harmless and regulators do not ask for proof of safety or efficacy. This lack of knowledge surrounding traditional herbal medicines, combined with an explosion in their use, demanded further investigation, and I was interested that Anusha's response was based on modern Western science, informed by an understanding of Indian tradition.

She explained this to me when we met over a cappuccino in one of Bangalore's many Coffee Day franchises, where we were joined by her husband and her clever, funny toddler, who was alternating her requests for cake between Tamil and English.

'There are some products that are not good products,' Anusha explained. 'That doesn't mean the Ayurvedic formula is harmful, but that the product could be adulterated. Ayurvedic medicines can be herbal, metal, mineral or a combination of those. The problems have come from heavy metal poisoning – lead, mercury, or arsenic. Even in chawanprash [a popular, particularly tasty dietary supplement containing honey, ghee, berries and spices and sold all over the world], there can be a lot of variation between companies depending on how and where they source the ingredients.

'The dosage that ends up in a product can become too high for several reasons. A supplier might gather a crop from a polluted waterway or next to a busy road, for example, or store it incorrectly. So now Indian producers are being regulated – herbal plants should be grown and harvested in controlled conditions. But the regulation still only covers products for export, not those for the Indian market. The other issue is how an Ayurvedic medicine or formulation is prepared. We know that the heavy metals which are used in Ayurveda can have severe effects, but this should not happen if they are formulated properly. When their use is described in the ancient texts, it's only after extensive processing during which they undergo a physical or chemical change that makes them safe to ingest. In this way, a toxic material like mercury can be converted into a medicine.'

By processing, Anusha was referring to how raw medicinal substances used in Ayurveda are first modified, for example by heating until red hot and dipping into a specified series of liquids; or by subjecting them to high pressures. It may sound a little like alchemy, but because what she was describing involved physical manipulation of materials, it is not unreasonable, scientifically, to suppose that those materials were themselves undergoing physical changes. How the original practitioners millennia ago thought these manipulations affected the efficacy of the medicines is hard to know, but using the language of modern science, Anu says that these processes of rapid cooling and varying pressures are techniques that would have altered the crystal structure of the metals. And whether a metal has the capacity to cause poisoning depends on these changes; its molecular configuration could determine how much of the potential poison is locked into the medicine or else is freely available to cause harm to the patient.

In her writings on this subject she concludes that even though Ayurvedic medicines containing heavy metals have been used for hundreds of years, their mode of action – pharmaco-kinetics and pharmaco-dynamics – are still largely a mystery that demands study both by people who are knowledgeable about traditional pharmaceuticals as well as by experts in modern chemical analysis.

This use of modern scientific language and calls for the study of the indigenous within the framework of the modern has long been controversial – both on the ground, from traditional vaidyas, and from above.

In 1947 the government-commissioned Chopra Committee reported on whether the indigenous medical systems of India could or should be integrated. The report concluded that the 'synthesis of Indian and western medicines is not only possible but practicable, though it will be time-consuming and not easy', and recommended that 'immediate steps should be taken in this direction'. Perversely, the government's response was that the theory and principles between systems were too different for integration to be practical. Modern scientific medicine was to be the basis for development in the new India, although the policy makers did concede that traditional medicine might also have a place alongside it.

Such duality was nothing new. By 1947, when my grandfather served as secretary to the Chopra Committee, he had been working towards integration of a sort for at least fifteen years. But it would be another fifty before the government of India would create a department for traditional medicines under its Ministry of Health.

At the time of independence, the general view was that neither the Western nor the indigenous systems were perfect, but that each had its own special merits and limitations. I heard similar sentiments repeatedly on my travels through India nearly seven decades later: that the 'valuable facts' provided by Western medicine – the precise details gathered from scientific instruments and verifiable empirical measurements – were offset by its 'poor ... knowledge of general principles'.

Anusha's husband Pari, an Ayurvedic doctor from Tamil Nadu who was studying towards a qualification in public health, told me how this use of modern scientific tools to deconstruct and study ancient methodologies still makes doctors trained in indigenous systems targets for criticism today. 'When you do studies like Anu's, people can either look at it like you're trying to make Ayurveda better, or that you are trying to bring the field into disrepute. But imagine if such analytical studies had been done two hundred years ago – Ayurveda could have been the mainstream now.'

Anusha had arranged for me to visit the nearby National Ayurveda Dietetics Research Institute at the Government Central Pharmacy of the Department of AYUSH, which covers the practice of Ayurveda, Yoga, Siddha, Unani, Homoeopathy and Naturopathy. I was to meet its director, Dr G. Venkateshwarlu, and his scientific officers. Anusha had told me that a great deal of government-funded research and analysis was conducted there.

On a corner off a busy Jayanagar main road, the 1970s facade of the government Ayurveda research building hid a wonderful courtyard garden filled with trees, shrubs and herbs. Along the seedling-lined corridors bordering the medicinal garden were laboratories and classrooms and we found Dr Venkateshwarlu's office on the second floor, at the level of the larger trees' branches. His office was large, with around twenty chairs arranged in rows. As he greeted us kindly, I noticed two large notice boards near the door which detailed the institute's aims and projects. Falling under the Indian government's Central Council for Research in Ayurveda and Siddha (medicine), the signboards detailed a résumé of the institute's achievements from its inception in the 1970s. I was particularly interested to see that its work on Ayurvedic formulations or rituals was framed in the language of modern pharmaceutical or laboratory research. The sign included details of a clinical trials unit ('194,657 patients treated to date'); a drug standardisation research unit, working on single drugs and compound formulations; a survey of medicinal plants ('26,943 specimens collected in medicobotanical surveys in eighteen districts of Karnataka'); and an ongoing clinical research programme ('Rasayana [a therapy for boosting energy levels, immunity and general health], obesity, dysmenorrhoea [period pain], and quality of life for cancer patients'). I also noticed from staff biographies that several had come from laboratory or academic research backgrounds: genetics, botany and neuroscience, for example. It was not what I had expected to see in an institution dedicated to Ayurveda and Siddha medicines.

I asked Dr Venkateshwarlu why it was important to the government that this kind of research should happen. 'In India, Ayurveda, has become alternative. The government is taking steps to mainstream this as a primary system; to move it from a traditional science to a medical science,' he began. 'The other Indian medical systems vary by place and traditions, but there are government Ayurvedic doctors throughout the country. Ayurveda can work really well with non-communicable diseases. In the West also, where communicable diseases are no problem, the issue more and more is non-communicable.'

'You mean things like obesity and diabetes?'

'Yes, and for malnutrition – eating the wrong foods – sometimes it's a matter of education. In India there are many people who don't eat vegetables,' Dr Venkateshwarlu continued.

'They don't eat vegetables?' I was taken slightly by surprise. 'In India?'

'Well, they cook vegetables, then they might dip chapatti

in the sauce, but result is they will eat things that make them feel full rather than balanced meals – high starch, fibre, but no nutrients. In pregnancy also, for example, to keep the baby small so labour will be less painful, women will restrict protein intake. We run health camps that regularly go out to rural areas to educate people about good nutrition.

'The origin of the [Indian] diet is medicinal. You know Vasco da Gama came, the Britishers came – they all came to take the spice, which was for taste, but also medicinal. Across India, people have adapted regimes ... traditional practices, regional, therapeutic diets. But dietetics is a neglected area in Ayurveda. The thing about recipes described in the scriptures is that it is not mentioned how much to take, only what to eat. Food generally, there is no dose, just satisfaction. There is no scientific validation for Ayurvedic diets [dietetics], so the government set up this research with the Central Food Research Institute and Institute for Nutrition.'

Dr Venkateshwarlu also described how they might tackle the problem of malnutrition, or other conditions such as gastric problems. He told me that after an extensive study of the active components of an Ayurvedic formulation for a disease, the idea was to come up with a dietary supplement. They might take wheat flour and enrich it with Ayurvedic ingredients. They were also using recipes described in the scriptures, supplementing staples like rice with them and dehydrating the results for use as a powder that would keep its shelf life and potency. 'We've already developed an antibiotic food formulation and a gastric formulation,' he said.

Unlike some of the commercially available formulations that Anusha had been concerned about, the sources of the National Ayurveda Dietetics Research Institute's plants – in their medical formulations as well as in their medico-botanical gardens – were evident. Opposite the noticeboard listing the 26,943 specimens from the institute's surveys over the years, the wall to the right of Dr Venkateshwarlu's desk served as a gallery for photographs of all manner of leaves, fruits, herbs and trees, labelled with their names in Latin and English transliterations from the Sanskrit.

'They come from different forest regions,' he explained as I surveyed them. 'Our researchers make trips into the forests four times a year. The teams are made up of botanists as well as Ayurvedic plant specialists. They stay for fifteen days, collecting plants needed for Ayurvedic formulations, doing surveys of the forest peoples – recording their folklore with respect to the plants. In this way we sometimes come across plants not used in Ayurveda, some not even known to us, medicinally. There was one we came across, for example, a Zamina – this is a South American plant …'

'And it was growing in a Karnataka forest?' I asked.

'It must have been brought in colonial times – yes, it had grown there and thrived and we discovered that the local forest people harvested the fruit – for nutrition, but they also say that it is a cure for infertility. So we record plants and information like this.'

'And what do you do with the specimens when they are brought back?' I was curious to know whether they would be analysed chemically to look for active ingredients that could be tested as a treatment for infertility. Thinking back to how people who habitually use plants as medicine used to venerate them, I also wondered whether Dr Venkateshwarlu had a sense of what the forest people thought about sharing the secrets of their herbs.

'The tribes and locals do worry that knowledge will be misused. But they are sharing their knowledge, you have to give them financial compensation and we acknowledge them in our publications. The knowledge will also be sent to the Forest Department. When the team return they do chemical analysis of the specimens here in our labs.'

A few days after meeting Dr Venkateshwarlu I was

invited to visit the Foundation for the Revitalisation of Health Traditions. I had been told that this research centre housed a very large database of plant-based products used in Ayurveda, Siddha and Unani medicines. But, more significantly from my point of view, it was also affiliated with a recently built hospital, in which patients had access to facilities that integrated both traditional and Western medicines. It was a little way out of Bangalore's city centre, part of the still rural but rapidly expanding developments towards the new airport and close to my home. As I set out with Amreesh, a twenty-two-year-old taxi-driver from my village, we talked about hospitals and healthcare I asked if he'd ever gone to an AYUSH doctor when he was ill. 'No,' he said, sounding a little confused. 'I go to the clinic. Everyone goes to the clinics. There are about twenty in the town.'

'Twenty? In such a small town? Do you mean private clinics, or government?' I asked.

'Private. There are different clinics for different problems and they charge different prices, so we go where we can afford. My wife had our baby at the government hospital, though. She went there because some family recommended a doctor working there. She had to have a caesarean and he was very good.'

I asked him why she needed a caesarean. 'The baby was big. Three kilos.' That was under seven pounds. I told him that three kilos was not a particularly big baby – or at least it wouldn't be considered so in the West. 'Well, it's not that big, but my wife was very small,' Amreesh explained. 'She was only sixteen. After the delivery, though, the hospital was terrible. She had to stay for a week – the sheets were dirty, the ward was dirty. Every time she needed the staff to do something they asked for money, tips. We don't want to go back there again.'

What Amreesh told me reflected many conversations I'd had in and around Indian cities – with everyone from manual labourers in tattered saris to auto-rickshaw drivers to security guards to people eking out a living in slums. When they got ill, it was the pharmacies, hospitals or clinics of the mainstream that would be the first port of call. Though the state hospital system was woefully under-funded, there were schemes to help people living below the poverty line, so that they could at least access 'Western' healthcare, however poor its quality. For those with a slightly higher income, there was a plethora of private clinics to suit different pockets.

I began to get the impression that the World Health Organisation's assertion that seventy per cent of the population accessed traditional treatments as primary care might really be reflecting usage by India's majority rural population. Put off by remoteness, poor salaries and lack of access to the modern facilities that middle-class medical students would be accustomed to, rural communities tend not to easily attract or keep MBBS (Bachelor of Medicine, Bachelor of Surgery) qualified doctors, instead being often better served by AYUSH practitioners. AYUSH institutions across the country have approximately 62,000 hospital beds and more than 785,000 health workers. One conventionally qualified doctor might serve up to 10,000 people in rural areas, so it comes as no surprise that the majority are thought to use AYUSH or medicinal plants to help meet their general healthcare needs.

Traditional medicine is, on the other hand, seen as a desirable add-on to Western medicine among the growing numbers of India's wealthy. The popularity of Eastern medicine in the West may also have led to 'reorientalism' – a resurgence of indigenous practices in their country of origin. The use of Ayurveda-based beauty products in expensive Western spas and retreats was being echoed among the well-off on Ayurveda's home turf, who are increasingly buying into a new glamour of India's ancient prescriptions. As one doctor I talked to put it, 'We do see more interest in Ayurveda when there's interest from the West.'

But at the other end of the spectrum, the reverse was true: I had heard from health workers that poorer Indians preferred to visit Western healthcare clinics. In a rapidly technologising nation that had recently launched its own mission to Mars, there appeared to be a move by those with little to leave the old behind. And, even though, as Dr Venkateshwarlu had told me, Ayurveda and its practitioners can be found all over India, I had heard from Ayurvedic doctors in Bangalore that it was not so easy to make a living from it, unless you were already a well-established vaidya to whom patients came by recommendation.

As Amreesh drove through Bangalore, I wondered what this meant for the thousands of students graduating annually from India's AYUSH colleges. Throughout the city, along wide main roads or in warrens of homes and shops of the old towns, the footprint of both the modern and the traditional was evident. There were makeshift signs on roadside walls displaying public health messages: *Touch spreads love, not disease*; *Donate your eyes*. I saw vans parked on the side of the city's traffic-clogged arteries, disguised as tents under reams of exotic fabric and offering Ayurvedic treatments for sexual dysfunction and all manner of illnesses. Medical advertisements were everywhere – from large private hospital chain and IVF clinic billboards to tiny haemorrhoid and fistula clinics to alternative signs hand-painted directly onto walls, like the one that read *German dispensary homoeopath for old inherited diseases*.

Fairly soon after we passed that sign, we found our turn-off and headed down a bougainvillaea-lined track that opened out into lush green fields, either side of which were the buildings of the Foundation for the Revitalisation of Health Traditions and the 100-bed research hospital belonging to the Institute of Ayurveda and Integrative Medicine.

The foundation had been established as a non-profit public trust in 1991 by Sam Pitroda, an electronics entrepreneur and technology advisor to former prime ministers

Rajiv Gandhi and Manmohan Singh; and Darshan Shankar, an educational theoretician engaged with traditional knowledge systems. The scale of their achievement is impressive, and between them, hold both the Padma Bhushan and the Padma Shri, two of India's most esteemed civilian awards for distinguished service to their country.

Over the years, their campaign to revitalise the practice of Indian health traditions has become widely respected for its standards of clinical practice and for its work in community health, as well as its significant contributions to medicinal plant conservation, the study of medicines derived from natural sources and products developed from them. The research hospital next door was started with the aim of reinvigorating India's medical heritage in practice, as a route to introducing a new type of healthcare that embraces India's main medical traditions – both ancient and modern.

Because Amreesh had been late picking me up that morning, by the time I arrived I was at least an hour late for my meeting with Dr Darshan Shankar. His building had been constructed in the traditional style of the Bangalore region, which would have been a common sight before air-conditioned condominiums and concrete-block housing began their ubiquitous spread. The environmentally friendly unrendered brick facade under high, pitched ceilings gave way to a cool, semi-open courtyard, filled with medicinal herbs and trees, from which a staircase led to the director's first-floor office. I knocked, and after apologising for my timekeeping, rapidly became absorbed in a discussion around the foundation's database, a mammoth collection of information on *materia medica* across India's systems: Ayurveda, folk, Unani, Siddha and the Tibetan Swa Rigpa. Darshan described how their database covered usage of plant-based medicines across an astounding 2,400 years from 1500 BCE.

'From my perspective,' Darshan said, 'we can see from the database that folk, Unani, Siddha, Swa Rigpa – they are all "expressions" of Ayurveda. Their theoretical forms are similar – and the materials even more so. If you query the database, for example, for plants used in Unani, you will find four hundred to five hundred indigenous Indian species – meaning that Unani probably absorbed India's *materia medica*, rather than bringing with it a whole other set of medicinal plants. When you look at the ingredients in some of its formulations, you see it's the same as an Ayurvedic treatment of another name. There has been a great amount of assimilation [into Ayurveda] – Buddhist, Jain, Islamic and colonial influences.'

Darshan pointed out that many of the oldest medical systems incorporate a strong practical element, but what sets Ayurveda apart is that it had a pre-existing, robust body of theory as well, cementing its status in India. 'Ayurveda is *so* important in India, other systems will find a way of talking through its language and materials.'

'What about the "other" using the language of bio-medicine: modern science?' I asked. I was curious about how much integration – scientific, theoretical and clinical – had already occurred and what Darshan's vision was for the future.

'You know, I had a cardiac condition six months ago. My family decided I should be opened up. So I went to an allopathic [conventional] doctor. He said to me, "I know what job you do – don't mix up all these types of medicines. Leave it to us." He said Ayurveda can do nothing. But now, post-surgery I am using a combination of allopathy and Ayurveda. OK, allopathic drugs can control cholesterol levels. But why do I have high cholesterol? We need also to look at the causes of that. Allopathy – biomedicine – is interested in maintaining problems within their limits, but the best of Ayurveda is telling me cardiovascular disease is a metabolic disorder. The mind is also a very important thing – I am also doing yoga for other reasons. Sooner or later, I *will* drop the allopathy.'

I was surprised that Darshan had had heart surgery so recently. He came across as being very healthy. He was slim, he looked well and he was full of enthusiasm and energy.

'Pluralistic choices have set the stage for people to ask questions and take different options when no one system has the answers,' he continued, 'but educational and health-care institutes have not caught up. Forty to seventy per cent of people are exercising that choice, the World Health Organisation report on the use of traditional medicines shows that. I'm not talking about practitioners, but for the public – sometimes they are well informed, sometimes they are not. So sometimes there will be good outcomes, sometimes not. In a nutshell, today, for whatever political and sociological reasons, Western knowledge systems are dominant in all parts of the world. So you have a system prevailing in Asia, Africa, Europe, America – everywhere – where Western traditions dominate. Its strength is that Western science has incredible knowledge of detail – the fundamental units of the physical world, *but* you don't have a picture of the whole.'

I was interested (though, with my geneticist's hat on, unconvinced) to hear from Darshan that in 2003, an Indian scientist, Professor Bhushan Patwardan classified a random population based on an Ayurvedic schematic and he showed that the three *doshas* (bodily constitutions) cor-responded with specific genotypes (genetic compositions). 'For us,' Darshan told me, 'this has opened the doorway to pharmacogenomics [the role of genetics in drug response] – it is known now as Ayugenomics. But Ayurveda doesn't need to do research in the same way as modern science. We are not testing a drug, we are testing a system of diagnosis and treatment.

'Such testing has been going on at least since the 1970s, when there was a study on the management of rheuma-toid arthritis in Coimbatore, in Tamil Nadu. Ayurveda is known to be efficient in the management of this disease. The musician Ravi Shankar had participated in the study when the condition meant he could no longer play the sitar and in a few months he was cured. But the 1970s trials designed by World Health Organisation scientists aimed only to assess one narrow measure of success: to decide whether the Ayurvedic treatment did or did not work. The Ayurvedic doctor in Coimbatore said that he would have used fifty measures. The trial was abandoned as unworkable, but in 2011 the University of California, Los Angeles came back to repeat the study, testing Ayurvedic management against the best allopathic drug, methotrexate, in a well-designed study. They found that outcomes were the same under both systems, but there were fewer side effects with Ayurveda. So there is now a framework available to counter reductionist designs of conventional clinical trials. We don't test only one parameter.

'See, it costs millions of US dollars to do biomedical research,' said Darshan. 'But Ayurveda has survived for centuries and was created by a long history, not by science. There are 5,000 medical manuscripts in Siddha, there are 100,000 in Ayurveda, covering aspects of medicine and surgery. It's highly, highly sophisticated. What Ayurveda needs to progress is to use modern tools. So the way we are working now is like this – the theory will be Ayurveda, the tools will be modern. And traditional theory must also grow in parallel otherwise it will lose its autonomy. If Ayurveda wants to come out of its marginalisation, today I have no option but to talk to the dominant medical system. In the future, in this age, we should be able to use modern methods to detect *kapha*, *vāta* and *pitta doshas* on a cellular level.'

I left to talk to some of Dr Shankar's research scientists, visit their botanical gardens and investigate the thriving integrated medicine hospital across the way. I thought, on the short walk over, about the point Darshan had made and what this would mean for the future of Ayurveda in India. In order to compete with the dominant 'allopathic' system, as he believes it is necessary to do, India's traditional systems require a different level of understanding and the development of new characteristics. While knowledge of its foundations will remain necessary, new applications of Ayurvedic medicine must see what changes are occurring on a cellular level, just as scientific medicine is doing. I was also very clear on what he thought the benefits of integration were.

'It is important to revitalise traditional medicine because of the marginalisation of traditional knowledge,' he had told me, 'for three reasons – because depressed traditional communities will get visibility; because patients will benefit; and because the frontiers of knowledge will expand.' Dr Shankar's thoughts reminded me rather of Hendrik van Rheede's comments over 300 years earlier. The demise of Ayurveda has been a concern for centuries, but it has always survived.

As I walked around the hospital guided by Dr Dhrudev Vyas, head of its operations and new initiatives, it felt like the realisation of a dream that had been sketched out multiple times since India's colonisation and after its independence. The hospital seemed strangely unlike a hospital: there was an air of calm and orderliness and a distinct absence of the ominous smells of antiseptic and disease normally so all-pervasive. Wards were comfortable and spotless. The doctors were a mix of allopathic-trained and Ayurvedic and there were also pharmacists, physiotherapists, surgeons, acupuncturists, radiologists, yoga experts and biomedical scientists to process patient samples. The nurses' stations, above which were signboards listing patients' rooms by the Ayurvedic diets their occupants had been prescribed, were manned by conventionally trained nurses and auxiliaries, sharply dressed in shirts and trousers.

On ward rounds, doctors both observed patients (by eye, for external clues and through biomedical measurements) and talked at length to them. Through questioning, they assessed the various dimensions important in Ayurveda for understanding what, for any particular patient, was normal or pathological function. Part of this was looking at the *doshas* (bodily constitution): – there might be an excess of *pitta* (bile, or heat), for example, but the patient's background – factors like their genetics, geographic origins and history of infectious disease – could mean that this make-up was unexceptional for that individual. One person's medicine could be another's poison.

Dosages, too, were very much tailored to the individual. Dispelling the popular perception that Ayurveda is slow to work, doctors at the hospital told me it simply takes time to optimise each patient's treatments because each regimen is personalised. Doctors also ascertain which of the patient's disease-causing imbalances might be be related to diet, activity and even the way they think. Without imbalances, they say, no disease can manifest. Equally, correcting a disease is not enough – success is achieved not when the problem the patient initially presents with has gone, rather, when all functions – sleep, appetite, digestion, metabolism – return to harmony.

Dhrudev himself had trained in biotechnology and microbiology and talked me through departments as we passed them. 'The integrative model is the key,' he explained, 'we have facilities for ECGs, radiography, a pathology lab: haematology, serology, microbiology, immunology – when patients have diabetes, we still want to know what their blood sugar level is. Our inpatients stay three to thirteen days typically and they come from all over India, as well as abroad. People hear about us by word of mouth. Even so, we also get two and a half thousand walk-ins per month.'

'So who comes here and with what conditions?'

'People come from all walks of life, all religions come, all communities – we have different price plans and subsidies. People below the poverty line will have up to one hundred per cent of their treatment paid for. We also run health camps once a month in rural areas – that programme was endowed by Tata.'

I had noticed that many innovative initiatives, hospital buildings and health programmes around India also bore evidence of the Tata Group's philanthropy. The enterprise, best known in the West as a steel company but which owns a multitude of business ventures in India, from hotels to jewellery shops to instant coffee and also counts Jaguar Land Rover and Tetley tea among their brands, contributes significantly to the arts, education, culture and health in India.

'You know, traditional practices have come into disrepute often because of bad practitioners, people who are self-proclaimed doctors. Other than rural areas, where folk healers are used possibly because they might be the most accessible, urban people will always preferentially go to allopathic doctors. So what you'll find is we will have people coming here for physiotherapy, rehabilitation, palliative care; after road accidents, cancer, or stroke. When there's nothing they [the allopaths] can do, we get a lot of those patients. We see many autistic kids. We also look after many patients presenting with stress or poor weight management; infertility, pre-conception, pregnancy.'

Dhrudev took me to the first floor, where the smell of fresh paint announced their new maternity ward, still being finished. Inside, he showed me the rooms for giving birth without conventional intervention, as well as one fully equipped for surgery, should that become inevitable. 'Because there has been a loss of traditional practice, people living in the city, away from their extended families – mothers, grandmothers – more women now don't have that support and guidance. We are seeing a rapid increase in caesareans in India now. That is why we are building this unit, so women can have natural, healthy pregnancies and birth.

'In this kind of integrated approach, there are a lot of good initiatives happening across India of late. There are some other places similar to what we are doing here, or there are some really top-of-the-range private allopathic clinics that have now integrated traditional medicine. There is a lot that Ayurveda can do.'

While the integrated approach might be revolutionising patient care, it might also have wider implications for the medicine across the globe.

'Over the years, India has indeed seen an increasing interest in its medical traditions,' Dhrudev continued, 'and in its sources of traditional medicines: plants and parts of plants, seeds and fruits for perfumes and pharmacy, Ayurvedic and Unani medicines sold in bulk and traditional medicines for retail.' In the mid-1990s (when Indian law did not allow agricultural and medicinal products to be patented), there had been wranglings with the US Department of Agriculture, together with US multinationals – famously over products from *Azadirachta indica*, the neem tree, from which seventy products had been patented. The corporate monopoly this threatened meant that neem-related patents allowed the holders to make major financial gains, while levying huge cost increases for the tree's traditional users. In India, neem had been used for millennia for medicine, toiletries, timber, contraception and fuel, and in agriculture as a pesticide and for the care of livestock. There were also legal challenges made over the genes of other plants, like nutmeg and camphor. Between then and 2003, the export of Ayurvedic and Unani products increased five per cent annually and exports to the US shot up from just ten per cent of total exports of these products in 1997 to an astounding sixty-five per cent.

I thought back to something Annamma Spudich had mentioned, about the low success rates of random search methods used in biotechnological drug discovery, despite the vast amounts of money spent on it. From her role as visiting scientist at Genentech, a Californian biotech giant, and from her days in experimental science, she had explained to me the standard procedure used to identify a new molecule that might potentially be beneficial in the treatment of a disease. It required determining the chemistry of a disease, sifting through vast numbers of randomly generated molecules created in line with that chemistry and then looking to see whether any of those molecules had an accelerating or inhibiting effect. But that random approach had not been particularly successful. 'A relatively small number of successful molecules have been found. It's really staggering, the amount spent,' she said.

I recalled that Darshan Shankar, from his Ayurvedic research perspective had also flagged up a similar thought: 'So it's important to go back to old therapeutic methodologies to see if there are easier or more successful ways to find solutions. At this stage in the history of the world we've largely managed to conquer infectious disease, therefore, the real problem is how to deal with chronic diseases. Chronic conditions are treated with single-molecule drugs and people are living with the by-products of these.'

In India, an enormous body of knowledge – centuries of records detailing what conditions these plant products are used for – are there for the taking. And now, with the comprehensive information on plants and medical traditions kept in databases like Darshan's at the Foundation for the Revitalisation of Health Traditions and the collections at the Department of AYUSH's Government Central Pharmacy, future foreign patent claims on the pharmacopoeia of India's flora may be easier to quash. Like the battles over neem products and the ever-present legal challenges and bans of India's production of generic pharmaceutical drugs, the dramas played out in courtrooms about medicines deriving from any part of the country's healthcare system has the potential to affect an enormous number of lives – both in India and in the developing countries that depend on her for cheap, accessible medication.

I had seen plenty of evidence of a concerted drive,

backed by the Indian government, to capitalise on traditional medical innovations that biomedicine may have been blind to. If it bears fruit, it is possible that the types of Ayurvedic medicine which will increasingly be produced for use in India and abroad will be single-drug formulations, closer to the rapid-acting 'magic bullets' which are a feature of Western-style pharmaceuticals: easy to test and validate in the conventional 'reductionist' way, widely preferred by patients and targeted at chronic diseases. Perhaps also, like Ayurveda's management of rheumatoid arthritis, there will be clinical studies more suited to the old ways, so that other traditional treatments can be tested and validated for adoption by both Western and Eastern worlds. And if these emerge, the integration of India's rich variety of ways to manage health and the bringing together of the ancient knowledge of plants and modern scientific tools may go some way to informing the quest that all patients have – to manage their illness, or to cure it – affordably and with the fewest possible side effects.

4

The Heart of the Matter

INDIA'S EQUIVALENT OF SILICON VALLEY began life in a town called Electronic City. Conceived in the mid-1970s, it lies around twenty kilometres south of what was then Bangalore's city limits. Today, the main approach to the heart of Bangalore's immense technology park is via a seemingly endless highway named after the Hosur municipality, just over the state border with Tamil Nadu. Neither the Hosur Main Road's multiple lanes, lined with hotel chains and Indian and multinational electronics corporations, nor the elevated expressway above it do much to relieve the congestion in either direction along its length. So the Audis, Land Rovers, BMWs or Porsches bought from the highway's many showrooms have little prospect of picking up speed as they are driven away; and every journey to India's biggest tech hub is necessarily a slow and protracted one.

Interspersed with the corporate headquarters and luxury brands were towns with a slightly run-down, albeit genteel feel, and it was near one of these – away from the main drag down a side street lined with fruit stalls and small family-run hotels and restaurants – that I found the entrance to another enormous complex, this one dedicated not to electronics or cars but to health.

Screened by a wall of large and aptly named flamboyant trees with their fiery red canopies, its foyer was surrounded by a wide porch topped by a double pitched roof of red tile, built in the vernacular style typical of pre-independence south Indian architecture. Rising directly behind it was a seven-storey L-shaped tower block, topped with an immense sign bearing its name, Narayana Hrudayalaya. In the broad scheme captured by the term 'Hinduism', Narayana is the member of the 'holy trinity' who protects life (placed between the Brahma, the creator and Shiva, the destroyer); Hrudayalaya means 'the temple of the heart'. Living up to its name, this world-renowned centre for cardiology (or Narayana Health, as it is more commonly known outside the subcontinent) is one of the world's largest heart hospitals and has, in the fourteen years since its founding, performed more successful paediatric heart surgeries than any other institution anywhere in the world. In addition to its staggeringly efficient output, the hospital has gained a reputation, fitting in every sense, as India's 'healthcare provider with a heart', because for over fifteen years it has been making world-class healthcare available to people who would otherwise have been unable to afford it.

As I lingered in the entrance porch, a little early for my appointment with its creator, cardiologist Dr Devi Prasad Shetty, I noticed that patients and relatives were gathered in worship at the hospital shrine, which stood in a garden just inside the front gates. In my line of sight was a portrait of Guru Nanak and an elderly man in a Sikh turban, offering prayers, and just past him, through its open window, another man, in his twenties, wearing a Muslim topi cap and sitting on a wall under an Islamic arch. Confused, I realised that what I had assumed was a Sikh temple was actually loosely divided into four parts: as well as the gurudwara and the mosque, under a dome with moon and star, there was a church with a Romanesque facade and topped with a cross, in which a lady in a sari knelt; and a mandir whose elaborate dome was carved with Hindu gods. That mixture of grief, hope, resignation and fear familiar to families of the dangerously ill was clearly recognisable in the eyes or postures of those praying in each quadrant.

'It is very important for the families, while their loved ones are being operated on, to have this shrine here,' Dr Asha Naik told me when she joined me in reception for a hospital tour. Asha, a former paediatrician, had been Dr Devi Shetty's principal administrator for the vast Bangalore health complex since it opened in 2000. Though she was pivotal to the running of a hospital that saw hundreds of patients and performed nearly forty heart surgeries a day on children alone, Asha was warm and almost languidly at ease. As we talked, she described the opening of the hospital, starting with just one building given to Dr Shetty to help him realise his dream of providing India with cheap affordable world-class healthcare. What had begun as a 225-bed heart hospital was now, just over a decade later, a 3,000-bed multi-speciality complex, including a general medical hospital with thirty departments and a separate dedicated, state-of-the-art cancer centre. The complex now covers twenty-six acres around Electronic City.

'At that time, this waiting room was very crowded with people,' Asha motioned to a very large hall, where perhaps around fifty to eighty people sat, quietly, in neat rows, waiting to be called into one of the consulting rooms surrounding it. Knowing the extent of cardiovascular disease in India, I had no problem imagining the room packed solid. Worldwide, cardiovascular disease accounts for the largest number of deaths not caused by infections: 17.5 million people die annually because of it. That's more than those who die because of cancers (8.2 million), respiratory diseases (4 million) and diabetes (1.5 million) – another disease which has also become a particularly virulent scourge in India. South Asians are genetically more susceptible to heart conditions than others, and it is projected that by 2020 Indians and Indian diaspora populations alone will contribute close to fifty per cent of the entire global cardiovascular disease burden. Of course, lifestyle factors such as lack of exercise and an unhealthy diet affect everybody, but genetically, Indians appear especially prone to their adverse cardiovascular effects and they also develop them earlier.

Heart disease is no respecter of class, and increasing numbers of the affluent have had to seek heart surgery alongside their poorer compatriots. The difference, of course, is that they can afford to be ill in style. Asha indicated a staircase to the extreme left of the waiting hall. 'The rich patients didn't want to come here because of the poorer crowds. We had to create a separate area upstairs for the wealthier people – the executive area. I'll show you later.' She smiled. 'But down here there are eighteen consulting rooms now. Dr Shetty's aim was to provide affordable healthcare on a large scale.'

The hospital's atrium was divided from the waiting area by an enormous stone carving of various incarnations of the eponymous hospital god. At its base, it was supported by a scene from the *Bhagavad Gita*, in which the Lord is portrayed dispensing wisdom and calm amidst a raging battle of epic proportions. In this spotless, marble-floored atrium through which hundreds of thousands of people have passed over the years were several reception counters: a travel desk for foreign visitors, a cash desk for taking payments, registration counters where patients were checked in and a dedicated 'Bangladesh Information' desk. This was to assist international patients from India's closest eastern neighbour: a less densely populated country, but one in which the people who need healthcare most face obstacles to accessing it as seemingly insurmountable as those encountered by the poorest Indians.

As I waited for Dr Shetty to see me, I read a fact sheet one of his assistants had given me detailing the chain of health centres that had opened across the country in the wake of the Bangalore original. Apart from the 1,000 beds housed here, there were now a further 6,500 spread across twenty-eight sister institutions in seventeen Indian cities.

The scale of what Shetty had managed to achieve in such a brief time was remarkable. India doesn't have anywhere near enough trained professionals to maintain the health and serve the sick among its 1.45 billion population, but the heart of the matter – the reason why Devi Shetty's hospitals stand apart from the rest of India's gleaming hospital-metropolises – is that they were created with a policy to be open to all.

In India, as in many areas of the world, the cost of private medical treatment is prohibitive to many, but the distribution of drugs and implementation of its public health programmes are also faced with massive bureaucratic and logistical hurdles, from endemic corruption to contradictory government legislation, which can make public healthcare equally inaccessible to the poor. A recent *Times of India* report detailed how, 'under the Central Government Health Scheme which covers central government employees, including serving and retired *babus*, current and ex-members of Parliament and the judiciary, the annual per capita expenditure is more than Rs5,000. In contrast, the National Rural Health Mission, which caters to the rural masses, spends just Rs180 per head.'

This is symptomatic of the inadequate regulation which sustains massive regional disparities and promotes commercial medical ventures while the public healthcare system festers through a lack of funding, the absence of compulsory health insurance, inefficiencies in governance and care, poor hygiene and low staffing. It's no surprise, then, that four out of five Indians choose the private sector, even when they can barely afford to do so. Shockingly, it is estimated that self-funded healthcare forces around 40 million people into poverty every year. Although the slick private centres are required by law to provide a certain amount of free care, in practice the legislation is often flouted.

Narayana Health seemed to offer a revolutionary new approach. As Devi Shetty put it: 'Corporate hospitals are developed for the rich, but also take care of the poor. This is a hospital for the poor and we also take care of the rich. That is why we exist.' I was struck by how Narayana Health had not only recognised the scale of the problem facing India's healthcare system but had also taken radical steps to change it – an almost impossible challenge.

Shetty had worked at London's Guy's Hospital twenty-five years previously and then returned to work in Calcutta as a cardiologist in a private hospital, seeing hundreds of patients a day but performing very few surgeries, simply because hardly any of the people who needed the operations could afford them. The experience spurred him to find a new way of working, in which efficiency, professionalism and skill would combine with sound economics to create a system in which those who could pay the market rate would do so and those who couldn't would be subsidised. Some criticised him for working outside the government health system rather than trying to improve it from within, but he was driven solely by an ambition to put world-class surgical care within the reach of people who needed it the most, and he felt that was a goal that would not be achieved via running the gauntlet of the state system.

'In India there are 1.9 million people not getting heart surgery; we produce the largest numbers of young widows in the world,' he said. Added to this, an estimated 78,000 infants born with congenital heart disease in India die every year because of inadequate healthcare facilities. This was a tragic waste of life from a reparable condition that was proving debilitating to the nation but whose treatment was out of reach to most who desperately needed it. In Shetty's view, if a solution is not affordable, then it is not a solution.

Built on land donated by his father-in-law, his hospital shortly thereafter began working closely with the state to provide financial assistance to poor patients through various means. A combination of government subsidies, fees from private patients and gifts from donors meant that everyone was charged what they could afford, even if they could afford nothing and irrespective of nationality. In India, it is not uncommon for families to refuse to pay for a baby girl's treatment, so these fees too were often waived. Those who are either subsidised or who are not required to pay, now constitute fifty per cent of the Narayana's intake.

With India's majority rural population in mind, Devi Shetty also created the Yeshasvini Cooperative Farmers Health Care Scheme, an inclusive micro-insurance scheme, now adopted by state government, in which poor farmers and low earners pay just over £2 a year to cover their family. Membership now numbers in the millions, though it is as yet only offered in Bangalore's home state, Karnataka. In the bureaucratic minefield of Indian officialdom, it must have been a formidable task to see the scheme implemented. When I asked Asha how they got the Karnataka government on board for these subsidies, she replied simply, 'Dr Shetty has great capacity of convincing.'

As well as the usual medical emergencies, some of the conditions eligible for treatment include dog bite, snake bite, drowning, injury from agricultural machinery, bull goring and electric shock, as well as labour and delivery, neonatal care and angioplasties. The Yeshasvini scheme has its critics, however, since it covers only surgical procedures and not general medical needs. There is a long list of exclusions – from burns and chemotherapy to spectacles and dental treatment – which, as the programme's metrics suggest, do deter a significant number of potential subscribers concerned about their more basic healthcare needs. Still, the small sum that millions of people now pay gives them access to approved, high-quality surgery (heart, brain and transplant surgery included) up to 1,000 times the value of their annual subscription as well as all-inclusive care while hospitalised.

One result of all this is that, in his home country, Shetty is now as close as it gets to being a rock star of medicine, adulation for whom, it seems, knows no bounds – in internet comment streams the words 'god' and 'sent by god' come up again and again. It made me think of the blurring of the spiritual and the physical I had seen in Dharavi. Certainly, to patients for whom any complex healthcare might have been previously out of bounds he must seem heaven sent.

As I knocked on his door, marked simply *Devi Shetty (FRCS, England)*, I wanted to ask him both how he had achieved so much, and why he thought other countries hadn't followed suit. I stepped into a large office where Dr Shetty sat behind his desk on a Herman Miller chair, wearing blue scrubs, a surgical cap and a stethoscope. As he fielded the various queries and phone calls that interrupted our interview, he radiated the sense of a man with a deep and peaceful centre, unflappable under pressure. At sixty-one, he looked ten years younger. Still, perhaps the wisdom of his years helped create the peaceful atmosphere at the heart of his hospital – its soundtrack was a steady, centring drone of a mantra, 'Om Namo Narayanaya' (literally, 'I bow to Narayana'); on the walls of his office were photos of Mother Theresa (to whom he had been first cardiologist and then personal physician) and Sai Baba; there were statues of Buddha and Mahaveera Jaina and a sofa for patients' families placed in front of a glass wall that gave Shetty a direct eyeline onto a lush balcony garden and brought its calming greenery into the room.

For a person who performed multiple demanding surgeries and would see up to eighty patients over the stretch of an eighteen-hour day, a base designed to provide some comfort and calm must have been vital – but the totems here seemed more significant than that. Shetty's space had a distinct feeling of sacred calm, appropriate to the hospital's Hrudayalaya suffix as a 'temple' of the heart. That he is proud of and dedicated to working for his country was clear from two national emblems on display in the room – the Indian flag and a model of the Ashoka Pillar that flanked a giant teleconferencing screen.

'I went to England for training in cardiac surgery,' Dr Shetty told me. 'In those days such training was not available in India because of the very small volume of operations. [But] I never had plans to settle down in England even though I had very good offers and opportunities. India is my country, this is where I belong and this is where my people need me. I am sure England is not missing me,' he joked.

But what if England was missing him? I knew that Shetty had already entered into partnership with one of the largest non-profit hospital chains in the United States to explore ways of using his model to cut healthcare costs in a country infamous for handing its patients the biggest bills in the world. To build and operate his proposed Cayman Islands healthcare city, the arrangement was for Shetty's group to provide technical input and running of the facility, while the US healthcare alliance group dealt with the purchasing, facilities management and biomedical engineering services. In the UK, massive government 'austerity' cuts to the healthcare budget coupled with growing migration into London and other urban centres, the stresses of managing an ageing population and staff shortages mean that, as counter-intuitive as it may seem, health systems of even wealthy nations might benefit from the Narayanaya model. Did Shetty agree?

'I strongly believe that all hospitals should be run as social enterprises. Because our customers are unlike customers of other industries: if they are not served then lives may be lost,' Shetty began. 'Primary and secondary healthcare [i.e. that provided by GPs and clinics] should be available at doorsteps of the patients. Tertiary healthcare [major operations] should be delivered in large hospitals where hundreds of procedures are done on a daily basis. In this way, the procedures become standardised, mortality and morbidity go down and the cost falls significantly because of economies of scale.

'Here we implant one of the largest numbers of heart valves in the world,' he continued, 'and, in the process, our outcomes are naturally one of the best. Because of the large numbers, we are able to procure materials at a lesser price than other hospitals. Again, because of the large numbers, when the result gets better, more patients come and you enter a virtuous cycle. This is the beauty of numbers.'

The next time I met him was in Manchester, where he was a keynote speaker at the UK's National Health Service health innovation conference. Joining him on the podium were Sir Bruce Keogh, also a cardiologist and medical director of the NHS, and Professor Gillian Leng, deputy chief executive and director of health and social care at the National Institute for Health and Care Excellence (NICE).

Devi described the methods Narayana used to keep costs low and increase efficacy – training local manufacturers to make surgical gowns cheaply rather than buying them in at high prices, for example, thus both reducing costs and providing local employment. He talked about the use of apps by doctors to engage remotely with patients who were unwell but did not need surgical intervention. Many of the doctors working in this way were women who would otherwise not have worked while raising their children. He described using text messages to keep staff informed and how hospital stays could be shortened by training family members to provide basic medical care at home – bathing, changing dressings and even simple physiotherapy.

'This is the power of not having money,' he told his NHS colleagues. 'When you have money in the bank, your brain stops working.'

Sir Bruce Keogh and Professor Gillian Leng were in broad agreement. 'We all have the responsibility to manage funds,' said Leng, while Sir Bruce noted that, when Devi talked about money, he only ever did so in the context of value. 'The problem in the NHS is that people don't know what things cost. How can we reduce spending if we do not know this?' asked Keogh.

He also believed that putting healthcare online, as Devi has already started to do, will result in a very significant shift towards putting patients in charge of their own healthcare. That, after all, is the direction in which the NHS also needs to head, if it is to continue offering free healthcare to the UK's growing and ageing population.

Shetty came from a very rural area in Mangalore, where the majority of the population work in farming or agriculture, meaning that they earn little but are extremely numerous. His vocation to provide free healthcare for all has clearly been shaped by his upbringing, and in particular by the chronic illnesses by which both his parents were afflicted.

'I guess that was why I became a doctor. My childhood was spent in fear of losing my mother. My father suffered multiple episodes of diabetic coma. The image we had of God as children was as a healer who could save the lives of our parents,' he said. Perhaps this explained the religious elements prevalent both in his office and in the hospital complex. In any event, this was an interesting thing to hear from a man who was clearly now very much a believer in God and who says that the reason he treats people in need for free is because it 'is the best way I can repay God, who has given me everything I wanted'.

Dr Shetty continued with his story. 'One day at school our teacher announced that somebody in South Africa had transplanted a human heart. That statement had a great impact on me. As a kid I was fascinated with the concept of using a dead person's heart to help a living person.'

The event he was referring to was the first ever successful transplantation of a human heart, on 3 December 1967, by South African surgeon Christiaan Barnard. It is hard to imagine now what a ground-breaking moment that must have been – today we think of organ transplantation as a complex, but routine procedure. To the fourteen-year-old Devi Shetty, it was a magical moment.

'That day I decided to become a heart surgeon. In fact, I decided to become a heart surgeon well before I decided to become a doctor. As a teenager, I did not have the maturity to know that I should become a doctor first before becoming a heart surgeon.'

Of course, even in India today, there are many young people for whom the ambition to become doctors like Shetty is alive and well. Why, then, was there such a desperate dearth of doctors in India today?

'Outstanding doctors have often come from deprived backgrounds, but myopic medical education policies exclude many potential candidates. Medical education costs far more than it needs to. After all, it is just an apprenticeship. Senior consultants train young registrars and make them great doctors over a period of time. But academics have made medical education so complex and in the process it has become absurdly expensive.'

The extortionate cost of obtaining a medical qualification is understandably causing a great deal of concern to potential students and their parents. True, to enrol at a public university is cheap (the equivalent of around £100 to £300, depending on the level of study) and there are no admission fees. But these courses are massively oversubscribed and competition for them is fierce. The alternative is to enrol at a private medical college, but that might cost upwards of £50,000, and nearly as much again in tuition fees over the course's five-year duration. And that doesn't include the inevitable bribes.

These expenses are unlikely to be recouped in India, where monthly salaries on qualification will only be around £3–400 in the public sector and perhaps double that in the private.

Some doctors find ways to supplement their incomes – by overprescribing medicines, for example, or requesting unnecessary tests. Stories of bribery and corruption are also rife. Of the rest, many leave for better-paid posts abroad as soon as they qualify, and most never return. India's elite All India Institute of Medical Sciences (probably the most competitive and difficult medical school to get into) sees fifty-three per cent of its graduates going abroad. In its cities, India has only around half the number of medical staff per thousand of the population that the World Health Organisation recommends. In the countryside it is worse, but government attempts to fill major care gaps – forced postings to rural areas, for example – have usually been met with protests and strike action: in 2013, nearly 300,000 medical students protested against the Indian Medical Council's ruling to make a year-long rural stint compulsory.

The West's gain through the medical brain-drain is translating into a loss that India cannot afford. The proposed solution is drastic: from 2015, Indian doctors heading abroad for higher medical studies are required to sign a bond with the Ministry of Health & Family Welfare that they will return home either after two years or upon finishing their courses. Those refusing to sign will be denied permission to work abroad. Some medical association representatives have complained that such a stipulation infringes on the basic constitutional rights of Indians. Others question why this scheme should not be applied to Indian engineers, scientists and other Indian-trained professionals as well (although, of course, there is hardly a dearth of those, and their careers do not in general oversee matters of life and death).

The situation may seem bleak at the moment, but in Shetty's eyes there is some hope, should India be able to force disruptive change. 'We are short of one million doctors, two million nurses and close to three million beds. If you start one hundred medical colleges [a year] for the next five years, that would result in a sufficient number of doctors by 2025.'

Shetty's vision is for a decentralised system of health-care training, where medical colleges will spring up across the country, in poor and rural areas as well as the big cities. 'Once they give preference to local students in the medical colleges, a small percentage of them will stay back in their own towns to serve the needs of the local population. This is the only way we can have equitable healthcare in remote locations.'

There are probably not enough qualified trainers in India to realise his vision, but Shetty has a plan for a global partnership to help with that too. Much as Narayana has been able to do for healthcare, Shetty believes that 'basic policy changes will bring medical education within afford-able reach of everyone'.

After leaving Devi Shetty to return to the ceaseless influx of phone calls and paperwork before his day's surgi-cal work began, I headed off with Asha to see how things at Narayana worked in practice. Our first stop was the oper-ating theatres. I was used to the idea of a surgical theatre as a hermetically sealed box, but here I found that, just like Shetty's office, all had large glass frontages with views to the gardens outside, which, the surgeons told me, helped prevent fatigue and the feeling of being closed in over the long hours of concentration that major heart surgery demands.

We visited the paediatric surgeons, one of whom, Shreesha Maiya, had previously worked at London's Great Ormond Street Hospital for fourteen years. I asked him what it was like being back. 'Here we perform about three thousand paediatric heart surgeries a year,' he told me. 'When I was at Great Ormond Street we did about five hundred in that time.' Incredibly, Narayana was producing these results with around half the number of staff surgeons as the London children's hospital. When I asked Shreesha how that was possible, his reply was, simply and with conviction, 'We just have to work a bit harder.'

As Asha and I continued our tour of the health complex on one of the golf buggies used for transport, I took the opportunity to speak to staff in some of its specialist facilities. We talked about heart valve donations and the valve bank the heart hospital had set up to support the thousands of surgeries they performed every year.

On the third floor of the complex's building dedicated to cancer care, I had a chat with Narayana's very friendly head of the Bone Marrow Transplant Unit, Dr Sharat Damodar. We talked about new frontiers in stem-cell science and I was surprised when he told me it was still difficult to get bone-marrow donors – in the West, donors of Asian origin are rare, but this was India. Even so, it sounded like there was still work to do in raising awareness among the public.

Down on the ground floor, a young radiologist, Rajiv Kumar, gave me a tour of their heavy equipment, including the three MRI machines that work until midnight every day to cope with the sheer volume of patients requiring scans. He showed me how he makes transparent plastic masks for patients requiring cranial radiotherapy in order to keep their heads still. I asked him about the types of cancers he sees – far too many, he told me, were related to smoking, or the chewing of tobacco, especially in poorer patients.

The expertise and dedication of everyone I met was impressive, as was their commitment to Devi Shetty's ethos of care. I got a strong sense that the workers here were vocation-driven, and importantly (perhaps because of this), they seemed happy, despite the immense workload that would-be doctors in Europe or America simply never encounter. The workstations of some displayed inspirational quotes or meditations on service and kindness. One postsurgical teenage cancer patient talked and joked with us as we came by. 'He said he put on his glasses,' Asha translated from his native Kannada, 'because he saw some good-looking people come into the ward.' As our golf buggy returned to the main hospital, I remarked on the warmth of the atmosphere Devi Shetty had managed to create for patients and staff. He was a very inspirational person – and clearly a spiritual one.

'He's a living saint,' she replied, entirely sincere. 'It's not only health and education; he has a wider outlook. See *all* of our drivers – these buggies and the ambulances and many of our security staff – are women. We saw many men doing the same jobs spending their salary on alcohol or something equally useless. Dr Shetty now employs women directly because when they are paid they save the money for their children's education, nutrition, their families, their future.'

Perhaps one of the most impressive things about Shetty is that wider world view. As well as the social impacts of his ventures on the local hospital community, on Karnataka state and on India, his philosophy is notable not only for putting low-waged or otherwise disadvantaged Indians at the centre, but also for expanding that approach to include the rest of the globe. Among the adoring comments I'd seen while researching this chapter were many from Africans, also pouring out appreciation for his help. The worship of Devi Shetty is a broad church.

On the ground floor of the cardiac wing of the hospital I was shown a long, computer-filled room, the focus of which was an enormous teleconferencing screen. This was the e-health unit, where technicians analysed patient data sent in real time from areas where there was no cardiology expertise. On the screens of the myriad computer monitors were graphs and metrics of the vital signs of patients from the deep, doctorless rural areas of India and beyond. Introduced as a pilot scheme almost immediately after his hospital opened in 2001, Shetty oversaw India's first efforts to deliver free electronic healthcare to the interior of India, where it remains difficult to attract any medical staff at all and harder still to attract the best qualified. From its site in Electronic City, Shetty's hospital served as one of two tele-medicine hubs for seven states of India, working with the Indian Space Research Organisation and Hewlett Packard for maximum efficiency. The first trials had resulted in the treatment of 10,000 patients in remote coronary care units, where basic measuring equipment can be sent for use by staff with only basic training.

'We do seven hundred tele-ECGs a day now,' the technician on duty explained to me, 'from the interior, but also from twenty-two countries from all over the world – there are fifty-three centres in Africa, many in Tanzania, also Malaysia, Thailand, Eastern Europe, Iraq. The readings come in within a minute from equipment they keep in the hundred and thirty centres and then our doctors process and analyse them here.'

'On that big screen,' Asha added, 'that's where doctors connect. We run eight training sessions a month, so that our doctors can exchange information and training with doctors from around the world. It's for their continuing medical education.'

The healthcare and education links Asha told me about were now part of Phase Two of the Indian government-funded Pan-African e-Network project – developed to share India's new affordable healthcare schemes as well as its specialist educational facilities with African signatory countries – Botswana, Burundi, Côte d'Ivoire, Djibouti, Egypt, Eritrea, Libya, Malawi, Mozambique, Somalia, Uganda and Zambia.

As much as Devi Shetty is an advocate for universal health, education and equal opportunity, he is probably also one of his generation's most dedicated patriots. As he has enthusiastically and emphatically said, 'We believe that India will become the first country in the world to dissoci-ate healthcare from affluence. India will prove to the world that the wealth of a nation has very little to do with the quality of healthcare its citizens can enjoy and we are going to do this within the next ten years. I have no doubt that this will become a reality, because this is the only way our civilisation will be protected.'

And I had no doubt that what Shetty dreams of, he probably will achieve – much as he has already done in a remarkably short time. It may be that Narayana's achievements have in part been driven by Shetty's remarkable charisma, but I also got the distinct impression that the kind of systems that he got moving just made plain, simple sense. Shetty has a very clear and precise way of thinking about problems. Concise in his speech and disciplined with his time, his skill lies in stripping away the extraneous and getting to the heart of the matter. He thinks of healthcare in the round, rather than its constituent parts. He had envisioned a certain reality and found the most logical route to get there.

The best solutions are often the simplest, but Shetty's brand of simple also had sophistication. His entrepreneurship is as hard-nosed as his personal ethos is spiritual, and his work is studied closely by academics, critics and admirers alike. His methods take into account what patients really need and what motivates staff. He has harnessed mobile health technology to bring diagnosis to places where no specialist doctors are present and enabled doctors to understand the economics of their own time, encouraging accountability by sending them daily breakdowns of costs.

Shetty aims to go to Africa when he retires. In the meantime he is trying to persuade a number of international educational establishments to set up a global medical university. He hopes it will train the massive numbers of medical staff needed in countries – India included – in which there are still simply not enough to go round. Rolling out solutions such as these, both in India and worldwide, is still a work in progress, but one that, if Devi Shetty has anything to do with it, looks destined to succeed.

5

Blood, Bile, Bone

I COULDN'T HELP WATCHING the reflection of his face in the rear-view mirror as Hakim Sultan Rasool carefully pulled a barbed thorn from his lip. It bled a little as it caught the skin and he flinched.

A few minutes earlier, he had asked our driver to make a sudden stop – one of many we would make on our early morning forage out towards the more rural landscapes outside Hyderabad, along roads that connected the old city with the new airport. This time, we had pulled up outside a one-roomed house, its once vibrant blues bleached over the years by the burning sun and and pristine whites stained by the monsoon rains. The front door was shrouded in a tattered curtain and, where there might have been a path to it, what looked like a grave covered in fleshy shards of aloe vera blocked the way. To one side was a low-growing cactus, its flat leaves bordered by spikes and flanked by an infantry of razor-sharp bristles. Hakim Sultan Rasool picked up a twig, wrapped it round one of the plant's prickly pear fruits and twisted hard. A sliver of a woman's face appeared, peering through the curtain. She made no objection to us being on her land and instead watched as he broke the fruit open and offered me a look at its oozing crimson flesh. 'The fruit is used to make a syrup,' he explained, 'for chronic tuberculosis. And I use Aloe in a formulation that works till second grade carcinoma.' He pointed to the 'grave'. 'After that it doesn't work though. But people don't know medicinal value. It's growing right in front of them, but they don't know.' He paused to swallow the pulp of one half of the cactus fruit and as he felt its sharp prick tossed the other back under the plant.

As we travelled on, the hakim, my Urdu translator Ramal Alwi and I passed littered undeveloped plots in small roadside towns, sparsely scattered mosques and homes and more wooded areas. As we went, Rasool pointed out the trees, shrubs, flowers, berries and barks he experimented with in his medical formulations. There were flowers used to treat rabies, the milky sap of leaves for the purification of blood, plants for jaundice, enlarged lymph nodes, palpitations, bronchitis, ulcers and first-stage uterine carcinoma. Occasionally, he ate a flower or leaf, 'Only because I know how to eat them,' he told me. 'Hm. This one is very bitter,' he said, swallowing it anyway. 'I recognise the plants by smelling, tasting and looking at their structure. In old areas of Hyderabad we can easily find these plants, but in open building plots being developed in other parts of the city they see them as weeds and destroy them. Here, in the rural areas, whoever knows about these plants as medicine, they will use them. *Har plants medicinal hain* – I think all plants are useful. Even if I show you some plant and say it is not medicinal, someone else might know what to use it for. I only take plants from here in an emergency, because they get polluted this close to the city. But see, in such a small area I've shown you, we've already identified nearly twenty medicinal plants. In the jungle there are hundreds. For my medicines I collect baskets full from the wild. Since I was eight years old I've been going out to the Warangal forests with my grandfather and father, I learned their formulations from them and I also experimented.'

As an example, the hakim pointed out another delicate shrub, growing close to the ground. As we bent to inspect it, he told me that its leaves are known to be useful in certain

rs. Based on that, and by experimenting with
ombinations of formulations using the plant,
able to help people who come to him with gonor-
and syphilis.

Does it work?' I asked.

'All treated successfully,' he affirmed. 'Effective *hai*. In one month the syphilis is gone.'

In India, 'hakim' is the title that doctors of Unani medicine (the 'U,' of AYUSH) are popularly given. As well as the decades-long apprenticeship in his family (of which he is the fourth generation) and with the other hakims in his five-year training at Unani medical college, Hakim Sultan Rasool used a large, beautifully illustrated volume of a 200-year-old text, bound in peacock blue and filled with painted depictions of plants and their descriptions in Urdu, that lay on his lap as we drove. The *Kitab Rehnuma-e-Akhakheer*, authored in an area of what is now Pakistan, was one of his trusted references: it details medicinal plants of the subcontinent and their indications, as well as their counterparts from other parts of the world – sometimes as far afield as Saudi Arabia and Greece.

The herbarium that Hakim Sultan Rasool used, and the medicines he formulated, were based broadly in a tradition known as Tibb-e-Unani: *tibb* being the Arabic word for medicine and *Unani* from the Persian word for the ancient Greeks. To India's close Islamic neighbours, Greece was known as Yunanistan and Greeks were called Yunani. Technically, the Arabic word *Unani* translated as Ionian – the eastern Greek-speaking people of Asia Minor, an area close to the island where Hippocrates was said to have been born. As well as being the name of the people, Unani was what their medicine came to be called on the Indian subcontinent.

Widely considered the basis of modern medicine, the theories surrounding health and disease in ancient Greece are thought to originate with Hippocrates, the fourth-century BCE philosopher/physician known as 'the father of Western medicine'. Hippocrates was from the island of Kos, just off the coast of Asia Minor (present day Turkey), which was the centre of Ionian Greece. Hippocrates organised the workings of the body according to the balance of four humours – crucial bodily fluids including blood and what he called black bile and yellow bile and phlegm. According to Hippocratic theory, any imbalance in the humours could result in disease and therefore balance was essential for maintaining a healthy body and mind. Although the modern 'germ-theory' medicine which eventually evolved after humoral medicine is – of course – very different, in some ways Hippocrates' understanding of disease was fairly modern, in that his diagnoses, in contrast with what came before were based on the idea that diseases had natural, physical causes, rather than supernatural ones based on evil forces.

Hippocrates' reasonably scientific approach to health wasn't adopted universally, however: fast forward nearly a thousand years to medieval Europe and you'll find a period lasting around eight centuries in which scholarship, education and literary pursuits largely disappeared in favour of religious instruction by the Christian church and scientific medicine had firmly re-dissolved into supernatural belief.

It would not be until the twelfth century that European medicine would develop again – though when it did, it emerged because of the existence of a vast wealth of texts written in Arabic, that had in turn been translated from ancient Greek. In 661 the Umayyad Caliphate headquartered in Syria (but stretching from Afghanistan in the east to Spain in the west and encompassing Georgia, Turkey, Cyprus and northern Africa) began developing what has come to be known variously as Islamic, Arabic, or Greco-Arabic medicine. The Arabic scholars knew Hippocrates as Boqrāt, or Eboqrātis, and honoured him as the 'first codifier of medicine'.

For around the next 700 years the work of Hippocrates, Aristotle and Galen were used and expanded, with learned texts filling the libraries and medical schools from Córdoba in the west to Alexandria, Persia and India in the east. During that time, philosophers, mathematicians, physicians – the scholars of rising Islamic culture in the Arab world – sought good copies of ancient manuscripts. These scholars also translated classical medical texts from India, China and ancient Greece. Reflecting the broad geographic spread and cultural centres of Islamic rule, many texts were translated from Greek to Syriac and then into Arabic. When, over time, some of the original Greek manuscripts disappeared entirely, the new, post-Dark Age European intelligentsia were able to benefit from the Arab translations of medical and philosophical writings after Islamic Spain was reconquered. There, in Toledo, European scholars gathered to translate some of these Greco-Arab manuscripts into Latin, the language of the learned in medieval Europe. In this way, knowledge derived from Arab scholars who built on Greek and Eastern traditions also informed the development of what became Western medicine.

But even before Europe of the Middle Ages turned away from the Greek model of medicine, there seems already to have been significant sharing of medical knowledge and healing plants between Asia and Europe, via the Arab intelligentsia. There is likely to have already been a long-running medical and scholarly exchange between West and East, between Egypt, Greece, China and India that might explain the ancient echoes of each in the others' understanding of health and sickness, anatomy and the treatment of disease. It is difficult to know exactly when this started, though there is archaeological evidence that by around the second century BCE, medicinal plants with an Indian origin were already in established use in Europe.

In 1974, archaeologists from Italy's Experimental Centre for Underwater Archaeology uncovered a shipwreck near the remains of the Etruscan city of Populonia, along the coast of Tuscany. The ship was dated to 140–130 BCE, a time when Populonia was a key part of the sea-trade route between the Western and Eastern worlds. It had been headed for Pisa or Marseilles, loaded with cargo from the East – glass cups from Syria or Palestine, pitchers from Cyprus, wine amphorae from Rhodes, ink-wells, lamps from Asia minor and ceramics from Athens. Its origin seems to have been Delos, a tiny island at the centre of the Cyclades, set in the centre of the Aegean. Delos was at the peak of its prosperity when this cargo was heaved aboard: honoured by the Greeks, Romans, Egyptians and even the Persians, Delos was the legendary birthplace of Apollo and Artemis, and in spite of its minuscule size (less than three and a half square kilometres), at that period in time its 25,000 inhabitants lived in a hub of international commerce, at the epicentre of the Mediterranean slave trade.

A thriving population of that size would have needed many doctors, one of whom might even have been aboard the ill-fated ship: among the cargo lay a range of ancient professional medical equipment, including an iron probe and a bronze vessel for bloodletting or pain relief, and something even more remarkable and rare: hundreds of tin and wood pyxides – small cylindrical vials – were found close to what had been a locked box. This too may have belonged to the ship's doctor and was perhaps his medicine chest, because inside one of the tin pyxides were five tablets, some still miraculously dry after 2,000 years of submersion. Chemical tests showed that among their ingredients were high levels of zinc compounds, known to have been used to treat disease in ancient times. The samples were then sent to a geneticist– who was sceptical, at first, that any intact plant DNA would have survived. But it had survived, and it later emerged that the DNA identified in the pills belonged to radish, celery, wild onion, oak, cabbage, alfalfa, carrot, yarrow and hibiscus.

These were all plants described in early Greek medical texts – including those attributed to Hippocrates – as ingredients used to treat gastrointestinal disorders, as well as a host of other conditions. The first-century Greek physician Dioscorides (whose *De Materia Medica* had been translated into Arabic by Ibn Juljul in Córdoba) described wild carrot as a diuretic used to treat colic, wounds and poisonous bites. Yarrow, which stops bleeding, was, mythology tells us, the same plant the legendary hero Achilles used on the bleeding wounds of his soldiers. And from tracing its genetic ancestry it looked as though the hibiscus in the tablets might have originated in India. Dioscorides' volumes on herbal medicines, written between the years CE 50 and 70, also listed other plants specifically marked as originating in India and detailing their uses as medicines in the Greek corpus, including: cardamom, spikenard (a valerian relative), cinnamon ointment, incense (*kostos*), agarwood, a myrrh-like resin called bdellium, aloe and *indikon*, or indigo from Indian reeds.

Well before Dioscorides' time, and certainly by 140 BCE, India had, of course, long made contact with Greece. Alexander the Great had arrived with his armies around 200 years before that; as a result, the Indo-Greek Bactrian kingdom annexed Taxila – a university town in the Punjab that was internationally renowned for its medical school. Under the reign of Emperor Ashoka, who ruled over almost all of the subcontinent between the years 269 and 232 BCE, famous rock edicts were commissioned to detail the emperor's provision of hospitals and medical treatment (along with public health initiatives such as wells and trees) for both humans and animals within his domains. These extended from parts of present-day Iran and Afghanistan into India's east and deep south. But he also delivered these 'among the people beyond the borders', as far as the southwestern seaboard (Kerala), into south India and further on to Sri Lanka, as well as to the dominions of Antiochus

Soter 'the Greek King', whose lands bordered Ashoka's in the east and continued to Syria and Turkey in the west.

Lost when some of the carved stone edicts were smashed over the millennia, the names and dominions of three further foreign monarchs with whom Ashoka had influence are now unknown, with the only surviving remnant naming one of the Ptolemies of Egypt, thought to be Ptolemy II Philadelphus, whose lands included parts of Egypt, Palestine, Lebanon, Turkey and Greece. As well as medical knowledge, Ashoka also stated in his edict that 'Wherever medical herbs suitable for humans or animals are not available, I have had them imported and grown.' The likelihood is that the sharing of medicines across a broad geographic region that included parts of the Greek world also meant the sharing of medical knowledge and expertise between East and West. Through the transitions of emperors and gods, conquests and cultural assimilation, this tradition of knowledge exchange dating back millennia saw a direct continuum into the religious and political flux of Hyderabad in the Middle Ages.

Historically at the centre of the global diamond and pearl trade, Hyderabad, where Hakim Sultan Rasool was born and trained, had also long been a region in which cultures interacted – not just in architecture, music and poetry, but also in sciences and medicine. After its conquest by the Muslim Bahmani Sultanate in 1347, Hyderabad prospered through a peaceful co-habitation between the original inhabitants and settlers of Persian, Turk and Arab origin. The city's rulers and royal sponsors fostered an environment in which Unani continued to grow and develop in conversation with local Ayurvedic doctors, incorporating the indigenous herbal plants they used. The exchange was by then no longer novel, as there are records of Ayurvedic scholars spending time in Iraq at the invitation of the Abbasid Caliphate in the eighth and ninth centuries; one, known as Manka, translated a key surgical Ayurvedic text while there, under the title *Kitab-Shawasoon-al-Hind*. Plants of Indian origin, such as sandalwood, had already been written about by the tenth-century scholar Al-Biruni and after the early fourteenth century, the exchange of medical knowledge in Hyderabad continued to travel in both directions.

This scientific tradition of exchange, experimentation and determining physical bases for health and disease is something that long-established hakims like Sultan Rasool continue to follow. Often, as his father, grandfather and great-grandfather would have done, his initial experiments were on himself. Meanwhile the Indian government's Central Research Institute of Unani Medicine, which has branches in thirteen Indian states, has since 2013 been conducting research using standardised clinical trial protocols – currently for conditions that include vitiligo, sinusitis, viral hepatitis, hypertension, diabetes and angina. The institute also works on scientifically validating Unani theory which, like the four humours of ancient Greece, is based on the idea of balance. Humours translates as *akhlat* in Arabic and Unani's humours are called *dam* (blood), *balgham* (phlegm), *safra* (yellow bile) and *sauda* (black bile). At the research institute, Tulsamma, a geneticist, told me of her project using the DNA of a thousand patients to try to understand whether their temperaments correlate with variations in their genomes. This would entail looking at samples of people all classified as having a dominance of one or other of the humours and matching that against information from their genomes.

Although the humours do form the basis of Unani theory and prescription, watching many of the hakims I spent time with in Hyderabad – as their unending stream of patients came in for fifty-rupee consultations through the day and even into the small hours of the morning – the traditional pulse-reading diagnosis I had heard of seemed almost entirely replaced by stethoscopes, sphygmomanometers and blood-sugar strips. The old methods of observing the patient's urine or stools are also now used in only very few cases. Cauterising and cupping, I was told, are time consuming and herbal formulations are used to balance excesses of *balgham* in the brain or *dam* in the body instead.

When I asked the hakims why treatment had changed, they invariably made the point that new tools do not belong to any one kind of medicine. 'Patients are all used to these kinds of measurements now,' Hakim Sultan Rasool began. 'I can diagnose from pulse readings, but I can't tell something like heart murmurs from doing this. For that I use a stethoscope. Normally, when a patient comes, first I do a differential diagnosis [to compare symptoms which may be similar in more than one disease, to determine which is most likely], to identify where there is pain or tenderness; which region, which organs are related to the problem. If there is something on the right, for example, it might be the liver, and if there is liver enlargement, is it jaundice, hepatitis?'

The patients who came from the large, smartly outfitted waiting room (predominantly women in black hijabs and jilbabs) into Hakim Sultan Rasool's intentionally tiny consulting room ('If it were large the whole family comes in together and then the patient may not be able to speak freely'), are here for both common ailments – sore throats, sinusitis, allergies, joint pains – and more challenging conditions such as thyroid problems, arthritis, paralysis, diabetes. In the hakim's mixed Unani and general medical clinic, one of three he owns in Hyderabad, his dispensary stocks his own herbal formulations as well as biomedical ones – simple painkillers and medicine for digestion, mostly. 'My patients come for both allopathic and Unani, they want both. Unani can cure diseases allopathic medicines do not cure, chronic conditions.' The hakim pulled out several tiny plastic pouches, each of which seemed to contain one small piece of gravel of varying size. 'These are renal stones. *Ham log treatment dey*, I have treated the patients who had them with Unani medicines instead of them having surgery. But if a patient comes to me with appendicitis, cases requiring major surgery, for carcinomas, I will send them to an allopathic hospital. I will use whatever is helpful to the patient,' he finished, 'because my aim is to make them better.'

After being shown out by his nurse, a girl dressed in a clean white medical coat from beneath which the vibrant colours of her salwar kameez and dupatta were desperately trying to escape, I set off to meet another family of hakims, this time specialists in bone setting – the healing of sprains, strains and other muscle pains, as well as fractures and full breakages.

As well as the hakims who deal in herbs and heart rates, there is another branch of Unani which had fascinated me for some time: the bone setters. I had seen itinerant street dentists set up their barber chairs and frightening array of sharp tools in the most unlikely places – under bridges, between market stalls – so I was keen to see for myself something that (for the more confident bone doctors, at least) would amount to street surgery. The one thing that doctors across India's state-sanctioned AYUSH healthcare system had told me repeatedly was that their treatments had no side effects. Not like allopathy, they would say.

Broadly speaking, the medicines that fall under AYUSH are seen by its patients and by many doctors as being natural and therefore risk free. This can be a very misleading idea, considering that any chemical ingredient that has an effect on the body – whether that chemical is natural or made in a laboratory – can always have related risks. After all, some of the most potent poisons known to man, such as belladonna, taxine alkaloids (from yew trees) or tetrodotoxin, are not laboratory made, but naturally derived. Still, when it comes to a type of medicine that involves not herbs but the physical manipulation of broken bones, there is a much more evident risk that it could end very badly in the hands of the wrong practitioner.

For this reason, bone setting theoretically operates under the radar within Indian healthcare, though in cities across the country bone setters offer their services to millions of people every day from their street stalls, windowless one-roomed shops and even specialist hospitals, some of which reportedly boast X-ray and MRI machines. In a roundabout way, India's government does support the study of this type of healing as a folk or traditional system that, if research could validate its safety and efficacy, might one day be given the official nod and be taught in Indian medical colleges. In keeping with its apparently relaxed view, not having a licence seems of no official consequence to the doctors or their patients, who appear to rely more on word-of-mouth recommendation. The lack of official status, though in some ways a boon for the bone setters, can leave them at risk of extortion by both criminal gangs and fraudulent officials, especially if they don't have formal training or state backing. But whether or not they can hang a licence on their walls, to their patients, many bone doctors are highly respected for their efficiency and efficacy, low cost and accessibility.

In the great breadth and diversity of Indian medicine, I had come across multiple bone-setting traditions across the country. These included families of bone setters of Fateh Kadal, Nowhatta and Hazrtabal in Jammu and Kashmir; Marma medicine in Kerala, which in times past repaired injuries related to fencing and their martial art Kalarippayattu; and more famously, a fourth-generation family practice from Puttur, a town in the southern state of Andhra Pradesh. In 1881 the first of their bone setters discovered a bone-healing herb by serendipity of sorts. While out hunting, Gopal Raju had caught a rabbit, breaking some of its bones in the process, and had wrapped the injured animal in leaves to take it home for the pot. But by the time he got there, the rabbit was able to walk, albeit with a severe limp. Suspecting the plant he had used was medicinal, Raju redesignated the rabbit from supper to his greatest experiment – he made a paste out of the leaves, applied it to the animal and reportedly watched it heal completely in a matter of days. (The herb is kept secret to this day by practitioners but has since been identified in a study by a taxonomist as Kasamarda, or *Cassia occidentalis*.)

Over subsequent years Raju experimented with chickens, calves and sheep, retrospectively incorporating ideas from Ayurveda's key text on surgery. The story goes that he then became part of the First World War war effort in India, when his services were employed by the British government for treating wounded soldiers and civilians. His brother's grandson, who had trained in general medicine, took up his great uncle's folk practice, opening a hospital that continues to be family run and is now one of two in the area, in addition to several smaller village clinics. Though the hospitals see more than 300 patients a day, the Kasamarda is still only gathered from the places in which it grows wild.

In Delhi and Jaipur the expertise of the *pahelwan* (wrestler) bone setters is well known, so much so that they must also contend with charlatans trading on the name without the necessary experience. Inside the walls of the spectacular city of Jaipur, many who specialise in treating fractures, sprains, injuries and muscular problems claim descent from the pink city's fifty-two historic wrestling schools, tracing their familial expertise to specialist knowledge developed by a direct ancestor. Among the bright and bustling streets of the old city, patients are bandaged and have healing balm applied in shops or at the doctors' homes. A few of these are romantically faded *havelis* – formerly grand courtyard houses often gifted to the wrestler by a ruler, which also housed the families' own wrestling rings. But when the princely states of Rajputana were formally dissolved after independence, courtly wrestlers in the newly formed Rajasthan sought alternative sources of income, making the transition from sportsmen to sports therapists. In Jaipur, almost all bone doctors produce home-made herbal remedies: in fact, rather than just physical manipulation, they say it is the knowledge of plants – committed to memory – and the ability to combine them that really makes the healing possible. As well as helping them to use formulations they find effective, this knowledge of plants, much as Hakim Sultan Rasool demonstrated to me when he selected leaves, berries and barks, allows evolution and expert experimentation to improve on what is already in use.

Many similar practices around the country are rooted in folk or martial and sporting traditions, but some bone setters do practise through association with what are India's codified, professionalised forms of AYUSH medicine – in Hyderabad, possibly particularly so with the Unani tradition.

As Ramal and I left Hakim Sultan Rasool to meet Hyderabad's most famous family of bone setters, we crossed the city's Purana Pul, the 'old bridge' over the Musi River. Behind us, the breathtaking Golconda fort of the Nizams of Hyderabad, with its curving stone turrets and old walls – once so splendid that they were covered with diamonds to catch the light from the candelabras that illuminated the castle at night – was receding into the distance. We drove on past bustling bazaars, romantically faded buildings along the perfect street grids and wooden shuttered shops, some embellished with ornate Saracenic arches and columns. We passed Hyderabad's most famous monument, the Char Minar ('four towers,' or minarets), which, with all of the drama of the Arc de Triomphe, towers over the intersection of four main roads. Still used by some as a mosque, it had been built by Sultan Muhammad Quli Qutub Shah in 1591, Ramal told me, to give thanks at the end of a cholera epidemic that had devastated Golconda.

Hyderabad's history was marked by the recurrence of these plagues: again, 300 years later in 1897 and then after 1910, no fewer than eighteen occasions during the British rule of India. The death toll was horrific each time – between 1911 and 1912 alone, nearly 17,000 inhabitants succumbed. In 1935, right next to the Char Minar and opposite the grand Mecca mosque, His Exalted Highness Nizam Sir Mir Osman Ali Khan Siddiqi Asaf Jah VII, the last Nizam of Hyderabad (and the richest man in the contemporary world), opened a large hospital dedicated to the study, teaching and practice of Unani medicine.

Unani clinics and medicines are certainly more visible in parts of India in which there are large Muslim populations (much of Hyderabad included). Its development through Islamic scholars under the early caliphates associates it with the religion with which it travelled into India; and yet even in those early years Unani had been in fruitful dialogue with Ayurveda, through Indian vaidyas who had been invited to the Arab world. In India today, as in the era of Hyderabad's rule by its Nizams, Unani is by no means exclusively used by Muslims, any more than Ayurveda is used only by Hindus. The Unani hospital the Nizam built in Hyderabad in 1935 housed 150 beds; but next door, he also attached an Ayurvedic section at great expense. Reflecting the contemporary importance of Unani and Ayurveda as well as the medicine promoted by the British, the building of these hospitals had followed the construction of a grand general Western medical hospital, boasting 400 beds and placed by the banks of the Musi. Like the Char Minar Unani hospital, it too had been designed in a splendid Indo-Saracenic style. Topped with onion domes and towers like something out of the *Arabian Nights*, the buildings are still magnificent today, but theirs is now a faded beauty. Although families like the hakims I met and unqualified street traders both run practices that are largely thriving, the investment from the state is insufficient to maintain the premises they use in their former glory. Crumbling plaster, paint bleached by the elements, damp and the neglect of underfunding are clearly apparent, and there are also reports of deeper infrastructural challenges. There are insufficient nurses and doctors, and years of neglect have left some wards unfit for use.

We drove on, past the rush of auto-rickshaws and vendors carrying imitation gold jewellery, sunglasses and plastic watches, sparkling sandals, pearls and brocaded bags. As we made pit stops to enjoy Hyderabad's famous street foods and its sights and sounds, I noticed that in this predominantly Islamic area of the city there were a few Unani pharmacies dotted around but no Ayurvedic shops. Though healthcare choices do not necessarily follow religious or philosophical lines, it was a phenomenon I had noticed in other parts of India too – the physical and spiritual are not easily separated.

Less than two kilometres from Char Minar and still in the old sector of the city, our car finally stopped outside an unremarkable row of shops. There, on a wall next to a furniture seller whose sofas spilled out onto the pavements, was the hand-drawn work of a traditional sign maker. Next to a drawing of a giant bottle of *lep* (herbal pain balm), there sported a cartoon image of a leg, fully bandaged from the knee down, and an arm, similarly bound from the elbow and encompassing all five digits. The sign outside the lock-up next door read *Hakim Gulam Rasool's R. Bone Setting and Neuro Clinic* in English, Telugu and Urdu, and below that, the names of the three practitioners there, 'Dr Hakeem Gulam Mohideen BUMS. *ortho – neuro and general Unani physician*; Hakeem Gulam Rasool (Babu Bhai) – *world renowned bone specialist*; and Hakeem Gulam Mustafa DPT (*Bone specialist*): *Spl. in: fracture and dislocation, spondylitis, slip disc, rheumatism, arthritis, bone growth, frozen shoulders, etc.*'

We salaamed, and before we entered left our footwear on the pavement outside – Ramal's sturdy sneakers previously covered by the hem of her abaya and the flimsy sandals I was wearing because it was forty-one degrees centigrade that day. The room, around four metres by two, with one side entirely open to the street, was lined with glass cabinets containing creams, splints made of wood and cardboard and stacks of soft, white cotton bandages. Hakim Gulam Mustafa sat cross-legged in front of us, looking a little bored. The clinic was empty but for his teenage sons, until the elder hakim, his brother Gulam Mohideen, came in to join us. He sat in one corner, beneath a wall covered in framed photographs of former patients and notable visitors to their practice. I found myself staring at two photographs in particular – both of young boys, perhaps around ten, with fractures so severe that their limbs had bent entirely out of place.

'That boy came in immediately after he got hurt,' Mohideen said, following my eyeline. 'The public know to come here immediately.' I looked at the 'after' photo of the boy's arm: well healed and back where it should have been.

Gulam Mohideen was the bone setter listed on the signboard with the letters BUMS (Bachelor in Unani Medicine and Surgery) after his name and was junior only to his father, Hakim Gulam Rasool. Aged forty-five and having worked in the family clinic since he was a young teen, Mohideen now ran a series of bone-setting practices around Hyderabad. Called Luqman Clinics after an Ethiopian former slave said in the Koran to have been given a gift of healing wisdom by God, the room we sat in was the oldest treatment centre. The newest (and largest) was to be a hospital on the other side of town, a modern, custom-built structure with an outpatient department as well as beds to accommodate inpatients. The other clinics had better provision for using modern anaesthetics, in which Mohideen had taken a postgraduate course. 'I am the only bone setter with a Unani and a higher medical qualification in Hyderabad,' he told me. 'I wanted to integrate anaesthetic injections to reduce severe pain.' Mohideen told me how in his father's heyday, until the 1970s, bone setters had the opportunity to apply to become Registered Medical Practitioners, or RMPs. In the days before AYUSH existed as an official denomination, this meant that doctors unqualified in Western medicine could receive legal sanction to practise within their systems, although they were not university-educated. 'But many people didn't know how or didn't bother, because, like my father, they had already been practising independently and developing bone-setting techniques for many years,' he said.

For Hakim Mohideen's family, many years actually meant nine generations. His father's ancestors had come from Delhi as royal physicians in the entourage of the Mogul emperor Aurangzeb, who, in 1687, besieged and destroyed Golconda, the fort about seven miles from Hyderabad, then thought to be one of the most impregnable in south Asia. That particular siege lasted eight months in a period of Indian history in which wars were a regular occurrence, with various battles fought between the Mughals, Persian, Indian, British and other rivals over the years. Battles – on the backs of horses, elephants, or on foot – meant injuries to soldiers, injuries that needed skilled doctors, working under the patronage of their rulers.

The financial security and freedom the trusted hakims were given allowed innovations in treatment to continue in the Gulam family under the reign of the first Nizam, who took over from 1724 when Mughal rule collapsed. The family knowledge of bone manipulation and bandaging as well as plants, potions and pain relief had been passed from father to son in a continuous line. In the small clinic in which we sat, as well as from the medical supplies in the glass cabinets, there were two large bowls of *lep* (herbal balm) placed on the floor, which were also part of that tradition. One was white, the other yellow. I knew not to ask what was in them – they are often closely guarded family secrets, made with ingredients that vary between practitioners. Hakim Mustafa described the basics to me anyway. 'The formulation of these *leps* are from generations back. The white *lep* is for massage; the yellow is good for pain. Its base ingredients are beeswax and oils, but for different problems, we will make different formulations.'

'All home-made. We don't market them so there's no certification,' Hakim Mohideen added. To his mind, as a BUMS-certified physician, bone setting was not an 'alternative' practice but one that fell under the remit of Unani, regulated by the Department of AYUSH. Hakim Mustafa described to me some of their other treatments, including 200 types of tablets, some with calcium, for example, to support bone healing; others, he said, would make the bone soft. 'People come here with every orthopaedic problem – fractures, also rickets, osteoarthritis, cervical [neck] problems … We open between eleven in the morning and nine at night, but if any patient needs me for bone fractures or dislocations after that, we attend emergencies also.'

The small room in which we sat was where everything happened, but at three o'clock, in the lull during the hottest part of the afternoon, it was empty. I couldn't imagine the small space bulging with the sixty to seventy patients I was told attended daily. 'There were less people coming in my father's days,' Hakim Mohideen said. 'The population is higher now. Everyone comes, now only maybe ten per cent speak Urdu [indicating an Islamic tradition]. We set the bone in seconds, but generally we spend fifteen to twenty minutes with each patient. It's not just the treatment that takes time. When someone breaks a bone, there is an imbalance of heat. Their lifestyle needs to be adjusted, they must have dietary restrictions.' Hakim Mustafa spoke more about the *akhlat* – Unani humours – applying Unani theory to conditions relating to the bone. 'People with more bile also have more heat – they are given a different diet – but only until they get well.' I thought back to the carrots, radishes and onions that formed the ingredients of the tablets found on the ancient Greek shipwreck. For Unani, just as for Hippocratic doctors, medicine starts with what we eat and is intimately linked with diet.

'There are more people in Hyderabad now than in your father's day,' I commented, 'but don't more people today go to Western medical clinics now?'

'For surgery they go to MBBS doctor. For every other fracture they come here,' Hakim Mohideen said. 'If they are poor people, they obviously come here. Even rich people come here if their MBBS treatment wasn't done properly. Bone setting uses movement during therapy, while allopathic treatment means patients need to also go for physiotherapy afterwards.' In such a system, the extra appointments required after the bone is set translated into extra expense that would have to come out of the pocket of patients – as do eighty per cent of healthcare costs in India. Add to that time spent out of paid work while immobilised in a cast and the costs of travelling to and from the hospital, and the prospect of going to an orthopaedic surgeon in the first place would simply not be a viable one for many patients.

'And what do allopathic doctors think of your medicine?' I asked.

'Doctors know us, they say if it's the Rasool family they don't mind. There are no other families here that have as much experience as us,' Hakim Mohideen told me. 'Without an X-ray, just by touching we can say whether it's a break or a fracture. But if we see that someone needs it, we will refer them to have surgery. For example, we do not treat injuries to the femur, because we simply cannot feel it well enough, because of its deep position in the leg. We will tell the patient, go to the diagnostic clinic, take an X-ray.

'There are people who set up as bone setters who don't know what they are doing. Sometimes we have assistants – people who hold the patient while we are locating the bone.

Some assistants look at what we do and think that it looks easy – they leave here and set up their own shop. But they have no experience.'

Just then, the afternoon lull broke and the patients flooded in. Hakim Mustafa, who was looking somewhat bored and disgruntled, burst into life as people arrived. The hakims, I could see, were passionate about their work – the change in the room was palpable as the first in line hobbled in with foot pain. He sat on the floor in front of Mustafa and the hakim methodically probed the foot with his fingers and thumb before pronouncing that a tarsal had been dislocated. Without warning, Hakim Mustafa gently pushed the tarsal as the young man's face tensed in raw agony for just a few seconds. When he relaxed again, seemingly at ease, he placed 200 rupees (about £2) on the floor in front of him as the hakim applied *lep* from one of the giant bowls, bandaged the foot and, with a reel of white thread, expertly sewed the edge of the fabric together.

'Patients come afterwards once a week for about six weeks,' the hakim said as the small room filled with people. 'Children heal faster; for them it normally only takes ten to twenty days.'

The next patient the hakim saw had turned up for his sixth appointment – a twenty-two-year-old who had been visiting Luqman Clinic every four days over the previous month. 'It was a total break of a metacarpal,' the hakim told me as he placed the man's arm on a large wooden block.

'How did you do it?' I asked.

'I punched my car window.' He smiled. 'I was angry.' The hakim asked if he felt better and he said that he did. He was no stranger to the clinic, despite (or perhaps because of) his youth. He worked as a personal trainer and his body-building regime had led to several minor muscular injuries over the years, but he first came to Luqman after jumping out of a window and breaking his wrist. 'I did go to the doctor for an X-ray,' he told me, 'but I had been told that these hakims were good, so I came here for treatment instead.'

In a brief gap between patients, my driver, who had been watching keenly from a bench outside the clinic, surprised us by stepping forward to seek the hakim's advice. He told us he'd been in a fight and punched a man, injuring his fist on his opponent's teeth. 'I did go to an allopathic doctor,' he explained, 'but he didn't fix it properly.' Hakim Mustafa duly did the requisite checks and treatments as Ramal and I looked on, hoping that his altercation and subsequent injury might have suppressed any residual road rage, at least for the rest of the day.

Even as the hakim finished treating our driver, the queue of patients was building up again and as the afternoon progressed, more and more of those in pain and those recovering sat next to us on the floor, waiting to be seen. A ten-year-old girl who had tripped down the stairs paid fifty rupees for her check-up: her pain had already diminished greatly after her initial treatment. An older man presented an ankle which was still bloody and scabby from a road accident two days previous – his regular doctor could not put a cast on the injury because of the state of the wound, so he sent him to the hakims instead, who applied fresh *lep* as well as an antibiotic powder under new gauze. Two veiled ladies came with a young girl to be treated; and then the hakim splinted and bandaged another woman, clearly in a lot of pain, whose loose chappals (sandals) had caused her to slip on a flight of stairs that morning.

I asked the hakims whether there were many women today practising Unani medicine. 'Don't women prefer to be seen by a woman?' I asked. The brothers told me that although there may be a preference for women patients, female practitioners were rare, but that when their hospital opens, they intend to train ladies to work there too.

As the sounds of the five p.m. namaaz began to be broadcast from the mosques surrounding us, Ramal and I rose to leave the hakims to their ever-growing crowd. As we did so, a young wrestler with a dislocated bone hobbled in. While Mustafa treated him, I chatted to his mother, who told me that as soon as it happened they came straight to the hakim brothers. 'If he went to the allopathic clinic,' she said, 'he would spend forty days in a cast and forty days having physio. I already knew he would be treated better here.' Apart from the prohibitive cost of seeing an ortho-paedic surgeon, being immobilised in a cast, of course, meant forty days of lost income – a choice that few people in the old city could afford to make. The young man, who had previous injuries of varying severity, nodded at what his mother was saying. 'Actually if I went to the doctor, this would certainly have been an operation.'

As darkness began to fall, the buzz of the old city, like the hakims we met, continued well into the early hours, when more of their patients were freed from their jobs and family responsibilities. I chatted with Ramal about my impressions of the doctors we had met and their treatments. The sheer volume of patients who by-pass allopathic clinics and go to hakims on trusted recommendations pointed to how far Unani was built into the city's social and historical fabric. Just as throughout its history, what I saw was that Unani, and bone setting within it, was still embracing and imbib-ing innovations from other systems of medicine sharing its space in India today. Hakims who blend the ancient science of Hippocrates and medieval Arab doctors with biomedi-cal diagnostics were evidently thriving. With clinics mainly placed in tightly knit, lower-income areas of the city, these doctors were very much acting as a first port of call within their communities. For these people who chose to pay hakims rather than the private sector mainstream medics (or opt for the free but generally avoided state 'allopathic' offerings), value for money was clearly an important factor. But picking AYUSH over Western medicine was not simply about the amount of money changing hands.

'That's the thing about Unani doctors I've studied,' Ramal told me, as our bandaged driver headed back towards her university at Hyderabad's Institute of Public Health. 'There's a lot of trust. Many of these patients actually do not trust conventional doctors. These hakims whose families have been in practice for hundreds of years, these doctors know all about their patients – how many kids they have – they know how many kids their kids have. They really know their situations and talk to them about their homes and their lives, not just about the injuries they come into the clinic with.'

6

The Fish Doctors

TWO MONTHS AFTER I visited Hyderabad's bone setters, I returned to its 'twinned city', Secunderabad, geographically separated from Hyderabad by the immense, sixteenth-century Hussain Sagar lake. I had been invited there by Dr Harinath Goud, the head of the Bathini Goud family, who for generations had been carrying out a curative ritual the details of which, when related to me by an Indian colleague a year earlier, I had found difficult to believe.

It wasn't just, as he told me, that patients came to the Bathini Gouds to swallow live fish whole; or that they came in their tens of thousands; or that the recipe for the herbal medicine the family stuffed into the fish's mouths had been a secret for nearly 200 years. As a unique phenomenon in India, what I found fascinating about this apparently bizarre mass medication was that over half a million Indians had received it in the last decade; moreover, the government of Hyderabad's state was subsidising the unregistered treatment almost entirely. The reason I had waited twelve months to arrange a meeting with the fish doctors was because the ceremony took place on only one day each year.

Unlike the old Hyderabad of the Unani doctors and bone setters, Secunderabad was largely indistinguishable from any of the recently built bustling neighbourhoods of Indian suburbia. Though it was founded by the British as a military cantonment in 1806, few relics of its architectural origins remain: its iconic 1860 clock tower only narrowly escaped demolition in 2003, having nearly become a casualty of the local government's attempts to ease the unrelenting traffic congestion. Other historic buildings were not so lucky. Just two months before my visit, a 400-metre stretch of old properties between the clock tower and the railway station were undergoing demolition to remove a traffic bottleneck and to speed up the construction of a new metro rail project.

The Kavadiguda area, where Harinath Goud lived, was an ordinary-looking place, with houses of no great age, general stores selling plastic toys and household goods and a few small shops stocked with snacks and drinks. There were no signs of great wealth here. I watched as an old vegetable-seller struggled to push his wooden cart into the street behind us. The neighbourhood bordered Bholakpur, an area which only a decade earlier had been the epicentre of a serious cholera outbreak. The root of the problem was its slum-like infrastructure: when toxic chemicals from the town's illegal tanneries corroded its water and sewage pipes (which were laid side by side fifty years ago), drinking water become contaminated and hundreds contracted the disease. Luckily, the outbreak was contained by the local hospital, but remedying the infrastructure proved more difficult. In subsequent years the administrative meanderings of the agencies involved had resulted in the sewage pipes being replaced, but the half-century-old water conduits remained untouched. In the same way that central Mumbai slums occupied prime real estate, so that shanty houses sat close to five-star hotels, here poor dwellings built on inadequate, unhealthy infrastructure abutted the multistorey luxury homes of the well-to-do.

But the Goud family were evidently relatively new to this milieu. The house we pulled up outside formed part of a new three-storey apartment block, painted pale blue, with pretty flower designs running up its height. The entire front wall of its ground floor was decorated with dramatic gold swirls in bas-relief and, like a family crest, a fish motif – curling into itself so that its mouth and tail came together in an almost perfect circle – was embedded at its centre. Although I had undoubtedly come to the right place, the home of the 'fish doctors', the gates were locked, and when I tried phoning, no one was at the end of any of their three phone lines.

I sat on their *thinnai* – a traditional raised, shaded platform between a house and the street meant for weary passers-by – and waited. It was to be a long wait and a futile one. In the three hours I was there, other visitors to the Gouds came by, including several young men who arrived hoping for 'passes' to circumvent the crowds due to turn up the next day for the medicine; a woman whose father had been successfully treated by Dr Harinath's fish and who had travelled 800 kilometres with her young family from Chhattisgarh in Maharashtra; and two of the Gouds' family friends in Brahmanic robes and priestly paraphernalia, who arrived on a motorcycle. All had fixed appointments with Dr Harinath that afternoon and I watched the increasingly familiar pattern unfold as they arrived, waited, tried phoning and left.

Those who knew the family were unsurprised by their absence. I was told that the Gouds were, as they were every year, at a temple close to their other address – a place in what had once been their traditional family village, now enveloped by the narrow lanes of Hyderabad's old city. The temple prayer ceremony was where their secret herbal mixture would be offered to the gods before it could be offered to their patients. Because their product was chemically unknown and untested, in recent years the fish medicine had been restyled as fish *prasadam* – something (often edible) that had been offered to the gods. In the same manner as some popular, off-the-shelf

Ayurvedic formulations; when referred to as prasadam this fish medicine took on the guise of a dietary supplement, avoiding any regulatory restrictions. This year, their gods must have taken longer than expected; either that or the family were stuck in the horrendous traffic that had been building all day in preparation for street party celebrations of the first anniversary of Hyderabad's Telangana state. I waited a little longer, tried their phones several times again, chatted to more of their hopeful patients and then decided to return later – something I was warned against. The evening's celebrations were predicted to clog the roads for miles around.

As I drove back, disappointed, to the university where I was staying, roads were being closed to all but pedestrians and a series of grandstands at various levels of completion were appearing along the banks of the Hussain Sagar lake. The speakers hoisted around them blasted popular music as we continued along the roads from Secunderabad and back into Hyderabad. Despite my determination to ignore the locals' advice, I realised that they were right – a return journey would not be on the cards that night.

The next morning I got a call from my friend Dr Nandu Kanuri, an academic at Hyderabad's Indian Institute of Public Health. Translating a section of a report published that morning in a Telegu newspaper, he told me that the Gouds' old family village was called Doodh Bowli and it seemed that the family would be staying there until the time came to hand out the medicine, which was scheduled, according to their astrological calculations, to begin later that day at eleven forty-five p.m. The exhibition ground loaned to the Gouds by the state for the event was in Nampalli, Nandu told me. 'That's very close to Doodh Bowli. So I don't think they will be going back to their new house in the next day.' Nandu and I decided that my best bet was to try to track them down in the old city. He added a couple of points the papers had detailed: that there would be a

1,500-strong security force at the evening's event; and that a crowd of 50,000 was expected.

The newspaper report did not give an address for the Gouds' home, which was understandable: I had heard of frenzied stampedes in past years and of attempts to get to the family that had ended in injury, or even death. If the anticipated number of patients was to be believed, it was not difficult to imagine the potentially lethal crush of those seeking the fish medicine. I got into the taxi Nandu had called for me and gave the driver vague instructions to get us to Doodh Bowli. Once there, we were going to have to be creative.

The drive took us very near to one of the bone setter's clinics I had visited two months earlier, deep into the old part of the city, down narrow streets where women in full purdah walked slowly through markets, men milled round the mosques, and children, oblivious to the call to prayer, chased goats that roamed the alleyways. On a main road a funeral passed, the cadaver just visible under its shroud, carried high by men who were taking it to the cemetery opposite. We stopped several times, asking locals if they knew the whereabouts of the Gouds' family home. Many told us that we would need to go to the Nampalli Exhibition Grounds that night, if we were after the fish medicine; others nodded in recognition of the name of their famous medical neighbours, but their vague hand signals told us to continue in various conflicting directions.

A man directed us down an extremely narrow lane leading to a maze of tiny houses, which occasionally opened up into small squares, or ran past formerly grand buildings and arabesque gateways behind immense outer walls, faded to sepia. My driver was sceptical. A short way down the road he asked again and a young boy confirmed the route.

'To the fish medicine house, you can go that way, left into that *gali*,' he said.

'But can we drive down there?' My driver looked worried for his car, which was nearly as wide as the road.

The boy assured him that cars did drive down the alleyway, so despite its precarious angles and the livestock and local residents who competed for a foothold along its length, we went ahead.

Where the alley finally widened into a market square, we stopped and asked after the Gouds once more. A tiny old lady, clad in a sari and with gold rings in her nostrils and ears, agreed to leave her vegetable stall and come with us as our guide. She seemed unsure about how to get into a motor vehicle, and a little uneasy once in it, but, true to her word and for a small fee she directed us straight to their street.

In among the predominantly Islamic homes, mosques and public architecture, the way she indicated appeared to lead to some sort of Hindu temple complex. A man urinated against its walled entrance, framed by a dramatic archway. At least sixteen feet high, it was coloured a vibrant shade of blue and displayed painted sculptures of Hindu deities, lotuses, conch shells, other iconic symbols and motifs. As soon as the car turned in, the temple came into view. With tall and ornate pointed domes, it was profusely decorated – much like its gateway – with painted sculptures depicting gods and goddesses and scenes from the Hindu scriptures, with enormous doors made of opulently carved wood. Inside, its elderly priest, dressed simply in a white lungi waist-cloth, held a burning lamp as smoke billowed from the censer he swung.

It was clear that our car would not be able to navigate the even tinier alleyways behind these walls, so I got out and, heading down a medieval-looking street filled with khaki-uniformed policemen, I found myself directly outside the Gouds' home, walled off from the street and with a red door that opened directly onto a family courtyard. Standing outside, answering questions and listening to the requests of patients who had arrived a day early, was an elegant man in his forties, dressed in a simple white cotton kurta and wearing a tilak of bright red powder on his forehead.

Still a little jet-lagged, I explained to him that I had landed in Hyderabad the previous morning after an 11,000-mile journey especially to meet Dr Harinath Goud, but that the appointment we had arranged hadn't quite worked out. The man introduced himself as Gauri Shankar, Harinath's nephew, and invited me to come back to their home that evening, to attend the prayer ceremony that was to take place before the medicine was distributed. I could then watch as the fish treatment was dispensed. 'Come at nine-thirty,' he told me kindly. 'We will talk more then.'

At nightfall, when the day's heat had abated to a relatively refreshing thirty-four degrees centigrade, I found Gauri Shankar talking to a group who had gathered in the streets outside his ancient home. The atmosphere seemed surprisingly calm, though from inside the doorway I could hear sounds of a crowd. Gauri Shankar whisked me past the house and through a door leading to his neighbour's compound. The narrow passageway opened up into a courtyard, around which apartments were assembled in the manner of traditional homes in Damascus or Moorish era Granada, or like the old riads of Marrakech.

I followed him as he skipped up a steep staircase, onto a terrace. 'You'll have to jump over this wall,' he said as he adroitly leaped from his neighbour's roof terrace onto his own. I followed suit, only realising the reason for the complicated route when I landed on a roof that was already filled with waiting patients sitting cross-legged in neat lines. When I looked down into his courtyard below, it was clear it had long since filled to capacity. The prayer ceremony was about to end and there was a celebratory mood among the crowd: I could hear throaty laughter and singing before, improbably, an enormous, cream-covered cake emerged to cheers and the refrain of 'Happy Birthday to You'. It was then that I caught my first glimpse of the elusive head of the family, Dr Harinath Goud. Bearded, in orange robes and with long hair, Harinath looked the image of India's traditional sadhus, respected men of God. The courtyard crowds previously seated now formed an orderly queue as Harinath and his wife, an elegant, jovial woman dressed in an orange sari, began to distribute the medicine. Many of the first to receive the blessed herbs seemed well-practised and I recalled hearing that those invited to the Gouds' home were neighbours, family friends and previous patients.

Giving the medicine out was not an easy process – the helpers of Harinath and his wife took an unsuspecting, finger-sized fish out of the container in which it swam, prised its mouth open to insert a small amount of soft yellow herbal paste and handed it back to the couple. The Gouds then instructed the patients to open their mouths wide in turn. Holding the wet, wriggling fish so tightly I wondered how they weren't crushed, the fish doctors inserted their fingers deep into the throats of those waiting in line. An inevitable chorus of gagging ensued as the living fish wriggled down to their death by digestion. For many of these second- or third-time visitors the process took just a few seconds and looked deceptively effortless – barely worse than swallowing an aspirin. For others, the procedure was clearly a far less comfortable one.

Feeling a little nauseous, I moved away from my vantage point to find that Gauri, who had been flitting between patients and making preparations for the queues now filling the roof space, was now back upstairs with me. I asked him about what was going on: what exactly was this medicine? What was the family's rationale for giving it and why did everyone (except, presumably, the fish) think that something apparently so extravagantly insane was a good idea?

I knew the medicine was widely supposed to be a cure for asthma, but I was having a hard time believing the thousands who turned up every year were all suffering from that one affliction. Indian herbalists and patients had often told me how a medicinal formula known to ameliorate one problem could also help with a host of others. Cardamom, for example, is popularly said to balance all three *doshas*, and is used to treat indigestion and stomach acidity, respiratory illness, high blood pressure and premature ejaculation. Or there is a species of wild pear lauded for its usefulness in treating asthma, dysentery, epilepsy, gastric disorders, menstrual complaints, lumbago and ulcers, not to mention as an abortifacient and an antidote to snake venom.

These were not easily dismissed as baseless claims: unlike many pharmaceuticals, traditional herbal medicines don't depend on one active ingredient. Instead, they use the whole leaves, bark or sap of a plant, consequently several active constituents may remain present in a single herbal preparation. It also chimes with the underlying holistic philosophy of both herbalists and Ayurvedic and Unani practitioners, of restoring balance to the body as a whole. However, few of these claims have been subjected to modern scientific scrutiny, so the evidence for whether single preparations might be effective for several maladies is largely anecdotal. There are exceptions – analysis of turmeric, long used in Ayurveda, for example, identified an active ingredient known as curcumin which was found to have a spectrum of biological activities: antioxidant, anti-inflammatory, antiviral, antimicrobial and anticancer. I asked Gauri Shankar about the medicine he was dispensing that evening.

'The medicine is for asthma, cough and flu,' he told me. 'Only this, nothing else. It has spread only by word of mouth [...] we do not make any ads. My father used to tell [us], in his day they used to prepare a handful of medicine. This year we are preparing five hundred kilograms. We are expecting four to five *lakhs* people (40–50,000). The medicine takes eight to ten hours to prepare and we begin organising one and a half months before. It is getting more expensive, but we do it happily.'

As the forty or so people who had been waiting on the roof terrace multiplied into hundreds, with more jumping over the neighbour's wall to join the queue, Gauri Shankar told me how his family found themselves at the centre of a rapidly expanding medical tradition unique not just in India, but in the world.

'We are the fifth generation in this house. Our family has been here since 1845. At that time this place was [in] the jungle – it was outside the walls of Hyderabad. Our great-great-grandfather was a man called Veeranna Goud. He used to sell toddy (home produced palm wine) and he was very charitable. Twenty-five paisa out of every rupee he made he would give away. At that time in Hyderabad there would be a lot of floods. He would buy food and blankets and give them to people who needed them. One sage, a holy man, had watched him doing that charity and blessed him. He blessed the water here. It is now our well – that is why the house was built here, because the well is here.' Gauri promised to show me the well later, once the crowds had abated.

'Using this water and some herbs,' he continued, 'the sage taught him to make the medicine we give. But the medicine has to be free. If it is charged for, it will no longer work. We still prepare this medicine using money from our own pockets. All our brothers keep twenty-five per cent of our income for this charity.'

To ensure they had enough medicine, Gauri and his brothers spent months in the forests outside Hyderabad, gathering the herbs according to the sage's secret formula, then washing and pounding them to produce the 500 kilograms of herbal paste. Apart from the practical requirements, they also make time for the spiritual – performing *pujas* (Hindu prayer ceremonies). These don't come cheap: priests need to be paid, offerings to the gods bought and guests – likely a large number – fed.

Neither Gauri nor his family had been what I had expected. The idea of asking patients to swallow live fish had set off my quackery radar from the moment I first heard their story. But I struggled to think of the Gouds as quacks: though it was unclear to either me or the wider world exactly what was in their medicine, they certainly appeared to have a genuine desire to heal.

THOUGH THE ANNUAL fish medicine distribution is one of its kind, the drama of the proceedings is something that might be framed in the context of India's growing phenomenon of television God-men and -women, astrologers and faith healers who also engage their mass followings in theatrical spectacle. Their power is evident when you consider that several have enough influence over their followers' minds so that some of them reportedly get away with engaging in excessive behaviour (ranging from the unsavoury to the criminal); while amassing large sums of money and securing the backing of politicians and the powerful.

But what's particularly interesting in a medical context is their marketing of health-related formulations to devotees whose ears and hearts they have already captured through millions of television screens daily. Television yogi Baba Ramdev, for example, is associated with the Patanjali company (which in turn, owns 90 per cent of a television channel too). Patanjali makes a range of consumer and food products promoted by Ramdev, including cornflakes ('cheaper than Kellog's') and instant noodles ('cheaper than Maggi's'); as well as Ayurvedic medicines for a range of conditions: including yoga for paralysis and hepatitis; herbal formulations for diabetes, weight loss, infertility and sexual dysfunction; hair oil and face washes which claim to help with dark spots and pigmentation. In 2015, their sales were reported to amount to 2,000 Crore (over 200 Million GBP or 300 million US dollars).

You might say there are some similarities between Gauri and his brothers and people like Ramdev: they are not qualified medical practitioners; their patients have no strong evidential basis for believing in their cures; they are educated, well spoken, and have the trust of their close community; and word of mouth recommendations and sheer force of numbers are also a powerful force in the uptake of their products. The similarities, though, probably stop there.

I knew better than to ask outright what was in the paste – the family would never disclose the recipe gifted to their ancestor by the sage. As Gauri told me, 'Only our brothers and their wives know what is in the medicine. Not even our sisters, because once they are married they go to another family.' I couldn't be certain, of course, but I did not get the impression that this secrecy was particularly a proprietorial move. With a medical practice this successful, imitators abounded and the family's website made a point of emphasising that if the medicine is not given by the Goud family and for free, it will be ineffectual. Revealing the herbal mix, I was told, would open their practice up to the market, to those who traded in healing and profited from it. And, as Gauri said, if the vow his ancestor had made to the sage that money would never change hands was broken, the formula that had been so effective would, by the holy man's posthumous volition, cease to work. But even if I wasn't going to be told what the paste was made of, I was curious to know the rationale behind their treatment, so I asked Gauri how it worked.

'There are some types of plants from which we prepare medicines,' he began, still naming no names. 'Every plant has natural steroids. The thing is, we need to recognise what steroids and what type of steroids. The medicine works because of these natural steroids.'

It made sense that a medication for asthma would be based on steroids: asthma sufferers worldwide receive corticosteroids via inhalers, or tablets or injections which mimic steroids naturally produced in the body to calm inflamed airways, helping to ease and prevent the typically asthmatic symptoms of coughing, wheezing and shortness of breath and also making it less likely that sufferers will react to triggers such as pollen or air pollutants. Phytosterols – plant steroids – are in the cell walls of plants and look and behave a lot like cholesterol. Practically every scientific study of plants used in traditional medicine for asthma has identified steroids as a possible active ingredient. Most plants contain at least some of the several hundred different sterols found in nature, including many that we eat – spinach, mustard, fenugreek, coriander and celery for example – and some will have more 'potent' sterols than others. However, the amount of sterols we absorb from what we ingest is minimal, and without knowing the Gouds' herbal recipe it is impossible to say what, if any, effect it might have.

Still, in very general terms of the science, so far so good. But then Gauri continued, 'The effectiveness of the medicine is based on the stars and on the time [at which it is given]. After the fish *prasadam* is administered, the patient has to be on a forty-five-day diet where they are only allowed to eat twenty-five items. We are not Ayurvedic doctors, but this medicine and diet is based on Ayurveda.'

I had read that the treatment cycle would officially end when the stars Arudra (Betelgeuse), Punarvasu (corresponding to Castor and Pollux) and Pusyami Karthi (stars in the constellation of Cancer) are in ascendance. In India, still today, marriages happen at times the stars dictate and to matches they recommend, babies are named according to lucky constellations ruling the time of their birth, buildings are constructed, journeys begun, space missions launched. To the Gouds, the mixture of the practical and the superstitious was also absolutely inherent to the efficacy of their prescription.

'And why does this only happen on a certain day and time?' I asked. I expected talk of the constellations falling into place, but this time Gauri's answer was a soundly practical one. 'This time is when the summer season changes.

The months of rain start after this. It is at this time that asthma gets worse,' he said.

'So why do you need the fish?' It was the star ingredient, the one that clearly set this asthma treatment apart from any offered in India's AYUSH medicine.

'When there is asthma, the airbags in the lungs will be having congestion,' Gauri told me. 'That, till now, there is no surgery to correct. No permanent cure exists – there is only an inhaler. The fish is alive, so it swims down the throat. While going through, the fish cuts through the phlegm with its tail. These fish – we only use murrel fish – they are very strong, fish flow against the current. Then they go to the digestive system, they get dissolved in minutes.'

It was interesting, I thought, that like anyone who produced medicines, from pharma companies to home remedies, it was always important to understand how these treatments were going to reach the area of the body where they were needed. For pharmaceutical companies, drug-delivery studies are complex affairs – if an ingredient is sensitive to damage by stomach acid, for example, tablets are covered in protective films or casings or are made soluble. For the Gouds, the living murrel fish was the drug-delivery system, forming a casing that protected their herbs and at the same time forcing it through any phlegmy congestion in the throat of people with asthma.

However, because of the anatomy of the passages to our stomachs and lungs, I was doubtful about the necessity of a wriggling, slippery fish. Past our throat area there are two 'tubes': the trachea (leading to the lungs, where excess mucus in asthmatics is secreted) and the oesophagus, leading into the stomach, the final destination of the murrel fish. All food, which is what these live fish would be recognised as, travels down the passage to the stomach, because when the mouth opens to swallow something, the trachea closes off to prevent it entering the lungs and causing asphyxiation. That means that the value of a fish powering through mucus applies only to a length of about ten centi-metres, after which, the fish will have a free run towards the stomach, with a helping hand from gravity. Moreover, some of the Gouds' vegetarian patients were given an alternative delivery system – an unrefined sugar paste called jaggery. The sheer drama (and, for many, trauma) of swallowing a live fish might equally have induced a placebo effect. The effort of its ingestion perhaps invoked an undeniable, vis-ceral sense in recipients that an intervention had indeed taken place and, therefore, that there would be an effect.

Murrel fish are grilled, salted and curried across South East Asia. A murky deep brown colour with fine black stria-tions, some species can grow up to a metre long in the wild, but mostly, as they are a farmed delicacy, they are eaten when they are rather smaller. Aside from their alleged phlegm-destroying abilities, it is this availability that makes them a good choice as a vehicle for the herbal paste: for around ten years Hyderabad's Fisheries Board, amusingly housed in a giant fish-shaped building in the city, have been providing finger-length murrels to the Goud family's patients at ten rupees apiece – this year, 50,000 of them. I asked Gauri how the government came to be involved.

'This happened since 1996,' Gauri told me. 'Before that, we got the fish ourselves. At the time there was Hindu–Muslim fighting going on in Hyderabad. There was a curfew. But people come innocent to this place. All religions came. So the government saw that and they got involved. We used to distribute the medicine just over there, where the temple is now. We donated that land.'

After 150 years, the fish treatment system that first began in the village home of the brothers moved to a sports complex. Seven years later, following an incident there in which a man was killed, it moved once again, this time to the Nampalli Exhibition Grounds not far from the Gouds' family home, where it still takes place today. State govern-ment sponsorship for the fish treatment was wide-ranging.

This year, once again, venue hire and policing costs were being funded from the public purse. Then there was the announcement by Chief Secretary Rajiv Sharma, which directed various other state departments to make the necessary arrangements for the event to run smoothly. These included the Greater Hyderabad Municipal Corporation, Road Transport Corporation, Andhra Pradesh State Road Transport Corporation (to provide buses to ferry patients arriving at the train station), the water board and, of course, the fisheries.

While we were talking, the treatment of the patients on the rooftop continued; it wouldn't be long now before the brothers would drive to Nampalli to distribute their medicine to the tens of thousands gathered there. I spotted a lady in a rose-pink salwar kameez who had been waiting for some time. This was not her first visit, and I asked her what it was like to swallow a fish alive. 'It must be hard for vegetarians,' I said.

She laughed. 'I am a Jain. It is not nice, but I think you get used to it. I'd say I am eighty per cent better than I was before my first treatment.'

Jains are well known for their vegetarianism and, in the pure practice of their religion, avoid killing even the tiniest of insects as they go about their daily lives, so she was pleased when I told her that this year the family were offering jaggery to coat the herbs. Next to her sat a slight, sickly-looking young man in thick spectacles. Like the Jain, who had come from Mumbai, he had also travelled a long distance from his home in Gujarat – a twelve-hour journey by train. The friend who had accompanied him told me that he suffered from severe asthma, but that after his second fish treatment last year, he was forty per cent better. 'For a permanent cure they say we have to come three years in a row. He has had these treatments, and for the last two years he has not had to use a nebuliser,' his friend told me.

Sitting cross-legged on the floor next to him was a young

woman in her twenties wearing jeans, a T-shirt and loafers. She introduced herself as Shreya, an educational psychologist who had come from Delhi; this year she'd flown, but last time she'd travelled over two days by train, crossing the vast distance from her home in the north to Hyderabad, the gateway to India's deep south. Then, she had waited three hours with the crowds at the Nampalli Exhibition Grounds but this time she'd called ahead, asking if she might avoid the crush. 'The herbal medicine is free,' she said, 'the fish cost very little, but the trip and accommodation cost me a lot: the travel, somewhere to stay. My brother came with me as well. So it's not cheap for us in the end.'

Shreya thought her problem had begun four years earlier, when she bought a carpet for her room and started noticing allergies and sinus problems. 'I saw you talking to him [Gauri],' she continued. 'So how does the medicine work, did he tell you? Is it Naturopathy? Ayurveda?'

I told her Gauri hadn't revealed what was in the preparation, but that it was plant-based and, as such, could certainly contain active ingredients of some description. Without analysis, it would be hard to determine exactly what was in there and what it did. The bright yellow colour might indicate turmeric, which is known to have antiseptic properties.

'That's true,' she said. 'They put their whole hand into your mouth to make sure it goes down so you don't taste it much, but there's also a bit of a wheat-like taste. And when the fish moves down my throat I also notice a mentholated feeling. I felt something went inside and already gave me relief; it felt like mint candy.' That made me wonder if there was perhaps camphor in the preparation as well. Because of their anti-inflammatory, antiviral and antibacterial properties, camphor plant extracts are used widely in Ayurveda and as a popular folk remedy for colds, flu and bronchitis.

'After two hours you can take water,' she continued. 'If you can control it they tell you to avoid using an inhaler for two to three days. And he gives a paper on what to eat for forty days – that diet is quite limited – tea, one fruit, rice, garlic and ginger, only *palak* (spinach).'

'That's interesting,' I told her. 'These are all considered "hot" or "warming" foods in Ayurveda and Unani. And fish, because it is an animal, is considered hot as well.'

The association of phlegm with coldness is also an idea propagated in Hippocratic medicine. Perhaps some of the logic of these ancient medical systems remain present in the way we connect cause and effect when we become ill today. For example, all of us will have had the experience of blowing our noses or coughing up an increased amount of mucus when we have a cold (so called due to its perceived relation to seasonal changes and the coming of colder temperatures, a perception reinforced by the hot home remedies used to treat it: steaming honey and lemon tea; a shot of ginger wine in a hot toddy). The Gouds' recommendation to take warming foods, then, fitted well into this system of thought and with the theories of India's ancient systems of medicine.

'Medical doctors would say that all this is a stupidity,' Shreya said. 'My doctor friend in Delhi says it is bullshit, and if I think it works it is psychological. So I'm keeping my inhaler in my pocket and coming here for the fish. It gives me options – last year, before I ever took the fish medicine I had to use my inhaler two or three times a week. Now it's four or five times in a month.'

'What about your family, do they know you have come here? What do they think?'

'This is India,' she said, and laughed. 'The family knows everything. My *chachaji* (uncle) has asthma too; he said he's too tired to come here but he's getting relief from yoga. They all know I just want to do something about this condition. Since coming here last year I am breathing in a good manner, sometimes I used to feel suffocated in my chest. I'd say it's thirty to forty per cent better now. Hopefully after this time it will improve even more.'

Almost everyone who had been lucky enough to be invited to the Gouds' home to take the fish medicine had tried the treatment before. They returned because they believed they had experienced some level of improvement. I found it interesting that everyone I spoke to tried to capture this as a percentage – however small or large they estimated that to be.

The crowds started pressing into us as the people I talked to joined the treatment queues. In an attempt to stay out of the way, I tucked myself in near the low wall of the roof terrace which overlooked the courtyard. I quickly realised this was not a wise move, narrowly avoiding being pitched over the wall by the unrelenting scrum. I began to understand how religious pilgrimages could end in tragedy and made a mental note to ask Shreya her thoughts on mob psychology, if I survived.

The queues became amorphous and less well behaved. 'How can you push in?' Gauri screamed at one man. 'You are a man, stay back! Let the children come first!' He called forward first the most sickly, then the elderly and children. '*Bismillah ir-Rahman ir-Rahim*,' Gauri recited as he dropped a fish into the mouth of the first in line, an elderly Muslim with a long white beard in a pristine white salwar kameez.

I watched a young man in his late teens retch as Gauri's folded hand entered his mouth. The slippery fish wriggled out of his throat and onto the terrace floor. He was made to try again. It was no easier the second and third times and finally Gauri held his mouth shut until there was no longer any danger of the fish re-emerging. Another man, older this time, also struggled as the fish got caught in his left cheek: Gauri closed his mouth and slapped his face, forcing the fish down the patient's oesophagus. A small girl, perhaps eight or nine years old and wearing a black hijab, cried desperately as Gauri gently tried to coax her into a second attempt, even after she had almost vomited during the first. Through her tears, she tried again, still sobbing, but calmed once the thing was done.

For what seemed like hours members of the wider family and their voluntary helpers administered the cure. It was work that required great manual dexterity and unflinching focus. The more fish that were regurgitated, the fewer people could benefit.

Under the blinding floodlights and in the heat and hope of the waiting crowds, the whole evening held an air of religious fervour akin to an American Evangelical healing service. But no gods were worshipped here; the crowds simply had faith in the Bathini Gouds and their deeply held belief that it was their duty to give their medicine to every last person who asked for it.

Over the years, Harinath Goud, the family's head, had publicly and repeatedly guaranteed a complete cure for any asthmatic patient, no matter how bad their condition, if the whole of their prescription was followed. But as the popularity of the treatment grew, so did criticism from the mainstream, sceptical at the lack of hard data and irked by the complicity of the state in such a bizarre practice. Threats were made that, should Harinath not reveal his herbal preparation for scientific analysis, legal action would be taken to force the state to withdraw its backing.

Neither event came to pass. Here, after all, was one ready-made way of plugging at least a small part of India's great healthcare gap, and this year the first government of Telangana had again taken the decision to support the event, despite fresh objections from the Telangana branch of Lok Ayukta (literally 'appointed by the people' – an anti-corruption authority that operates in several Indian states) that the herbal substance's efficacy was unproven. (No studies of benefit or harm have been conducted to date: of the herbs, the fish, the water they are kept in, nor any effects of swallowing them live.)

Three hours after I had arrived, and with around fifty

people still waiting to be treated, Gauri announced that their supply of fish had run out. I could see a mixture of confusion, panic and resignation in the remaining patients' faces. 'You can wait here three or four hours,' he shouted, 'or you can go to Nampalli Exhibition Grounds, there are more fish there.' A man in the crowd advised me to move quickly if I wanted to stand any chance of getting the medicine. As he sprinted away, I noticed Shreya still in a huddle of people standing at the back. She had avoided the most unruly queues, but her wait that evening would now be an even longer one. After the chaos of her experience last year, she was not likely to go to the larger venue, and after seeing the crush created by a mere couple of hundred people – not to mention my own brush with danger – I couldn't blame her for not wanting to take her chances among thousands.

Once the rush had abated, Gauri was back to his old self – perfectly calm, as if there had never been any shouting, shoving or vomiting. His sweating brow was the only sign of exertion, although with the temperature still standing at around thirty degrees it might just have easily been caused by humidity. He caught my eye and beckoned me to follow him, and we headed single file down the steep, narrow stairs to the courtyard. Under the staircase, opposite rows of photographs and paintings of the Bathini Goud family lineage, was the sacred well he'd promised to show me several hours before.

'You know how hot it has been – see the water? This well has never dried. Never in nearly two hundred years. This well was blessed by the sage and we use its water to prepare our medicine,' he reminded me. He'd been right about the weather: the rains were late again and my visit had coincided with an unusual late-June heatwave that had led to a spate of deaths among the vulnerable.

I thanked Gauri for his hospitality. He smiled graciously and told me he had to run. I believed him. For him, as for Shreya, the hundreds at his house would be as nothing compared to the tens of thousands waiting for the sacred moment at the main venue.

'I have to WhatsApp some people first,' he shouted to me as he rushed through the courtyard doors out into the ancient streets.

'Patients?' I shouted back.

'Yes, to tell them if they haven't got here, to go to Nampalli as soon as they can.'

As Gauri disappeared into the night, I headed back into my waiting taxi, still parked in the shadow of the Gouds' temple, past the Jain lady in pink, who was now in a very relaxed and happy mood. A toddler in his father's arms next to her seemed also to have forgotten the trauma of the fish, his tears long dried.

'Did you try the medicine?' she asked as I made to leave.

I told her I hadn't, but that there was nothing wrong with my respiratory system. 'My lungs are fine,' I said.

'Touch wood,' she replied.

'Home?' my driver asked.

'Nampalli,' I told him.

He did his best to discourage me – 'It will be chaos, madam' – but I asked him to go anyway.

Hyderabad became a different city after midnight – no crowds on the streets, markets emptied of their wares. The traffic had vanished and its pre-independence wood-carved verandas and parades of shops with their crumbling, once-white plaster facades looked more beautiful in the cool calm of night.

At the tented, decorated entrance to the exhibition grounds rows of patients still waited behind metal barricades; police guards lined the street and attempted to maintain order. I asked my driver to slow down. This time he spun round to look at me. 'You're not actually going in, are you? There are thousands and thousands of people.' His tone was almost pleading. I looked in as the car crawled past, at the lines of people who had camped there for days and the hopeful new arrivals, looked back at him and told him to drive on.

In India, a country that had recently launched a Mars mission (albeit, on a day thought to be auspicious to the red planet), a medical treatment with no known evidence-base showed no signs of being relegated to the past. On the contrary, there was a mediaeval fervour here. It had originated with a holy man and involved a spiritual blessing. I was sure that next June, the crowds would multiply even further. For any patient to really be able to make an informed decision about the health choices on offer, you could argue that it is important to understand whether, and, if so, how such medicines actually worked. Treatment should also be given in line with a diagnosis, whereas in this case, patients turn up to take medication for a disease they say they have. There are no checks in place to ascertain whether what they believe to be true actually is. If it isn't true, then what unknown conditions are going undiagnosed under the cover of asthma-like symptoms? What really is the origin of their coughs? Still, here was a treatment that resonated with the psyche of a deep-seated tradition in which, in the pursuit of wellbeing, there can be no real separation of body and mind. It incorporated diet and lifestyle. It was said to have no side-effects. It was offered with no expectation of payment, or gain from the medical staff. It engendered trust. It struck me that in developing healthcare for India, and indeed any nation, it would be wise not to overlook any of these factors.

THE FOLLOWING MORNING, newspapers covering the Nampalli event reported unprecedented crowds. Head counts put the numbers of visitors at around twenty-thousand more than had come the previous year. The influx of the seventy-thousand patients had also meant that the fisheries department miscalculated the quantity of young fish of ingestible size, and so thousands of people would have been turned away, their journeys wasted. But at least they left alive. A sixty-five year old asthmatic man who travelled nearly six hundred kilometres from his home in Belagum, Karnataka, had not been so lucky. At around one o'clock that afternoon, while my disgruntled driver was helping me track down the Gouds' traditional family home, Basavaraju stood in the long queue outside the exhibition grounds, waiting for the venue to open. He had travelled there alone, so when his asthma attack began, the only people who were there to take him to hospital were the police guards, who rushed him to Hyderabad's historic Osmania hospital. He was declared dead on arrival, and the next day, after a post-mortem, they handed his body over to his son.

7

The Mother Goddess

THE GADCHIROLI DISTRICT in Maharashtra State was a ten-hour journey from Hyderabad, the last leg of which was a long, spectacular drive over immense dried river beds awaiting the monsoon rains and along small roads flanked by beautiful, seemingly peaceful forests of teak, bamboo and intertwining vegetation. It wasn't just the distance or terrain that made Gadchiroli difficult to access. When I told my Hyderabad family where I was headed, they asked me whether I realised that I was going into a terrorist stronghold. The lush forests which are home to Maharashtra's Gond tribes also offer ample cover to the Naxalites, an infamous Maoist group of guerrillas – and are well known as the location of their power struggle with the Indian police and military forces.

As we passed through, the scenery along the road was serene, if at times desolate before the rains; shrubs and trees grew out of the vast, burnt red earth while emaciated cattle made their way through rice paddy past small groups of women in yellow, blue, purple and green fabric that billowed as they walked into the distance, straight-backed, water pots balanced elegantly on their heads. But signs of conflict were not invisible. In a small, very ordinary-looking village, we drove past the camp of a paramilitary battalion. Guarding its tall white turrets was a beautiful young woman, dressed in khaki, rifle aimed in readiness.

As the one small main road became enveloped by the forest, now not far from our destination, my taxi began to slow. Two large buses had stopped, one on either side, and as we passed them thirty or so men ran silently and urgently out of the trees and towards the parked vehicles, firearms in hand and faces unmistakably determined. 'They're plain clothes police,' my driver said, seemingly unfazed. 'They must have heard about a Naxalite sighting here.' He drove calmly on. I was rattled, and very relieved when we finally reached our destination among the trees, too late and too exhausted to do anything but sleep.

Despite the local upheaval, the place I was visiting couldn't have been more peaceful. Set up in the late 1980s to bring medical care to women who had none, SEARCH (the Society for Education, Action and Research in Community Health) was a hospital camp cum research centre, the brainchild of an energetic sixty-four-year-old gynaecologist/physician couple, Dr Rani Bang and her husband Abhay. I was there to observe their work on women's and infant health. At breakfast in the mess, I chatted with some of the doctors, computer scientists and postgraduate students who were working there. The society's catchment area included the general rural population as well as members of the Gond tribe – the largest tribe in this part of the country – which numbered ten million people spread across the jungles from central India towards its eastern coast. Its medical staff provide much-needed healthcare while its scientists gather and rigorously analyse data about public health and disease, working to create programmes best suited to tribal and rural lifestyles and medical needs.

The camp's new dentist, a bubbly young woman from Nagpur (the nearest major city, a four-hour drive away), told me they'd been trying to fill her post for a year. I told her it must have been challenging to attract staff to such a remote location. She laughed. 'Well, it's not just that it's remote,' she said, as others on the breakfast table nodded knowingly. As they went back to their offices and clinics, I was starting to get the picture too. The hazards faced by the medical staff are severe: if you Google Gadchiroli, details of the long-running, brutal low-level war with the Indian state fill the search pages: police gunned down or killed in bombings or by land mines; images of blood-soaked or dismembered bodies of those who had crossed or opposed the Naxalites.

When I met Dr Abhay in the camp's office, I admitted that I was largely ignorant about the Naxal issue. Abhay, a physician and public health expert, had been brought up in the same state, in a peaceful Ghandian community in Wardha, before spending the last nineteen years of his life living and working in a war-torn forest. I asked him about the dangers he and his staff face.

'We haven't had any encounters with them directly,' he explained, 'but they undoubtedly have a presence. To begin with, the Naxalites were supporting the ideal of egalitarian society, and revolting against unjust landlords. When they came, they were very motivated, they understood what Marxism was, what revolution was, though they were not very clear how they would bring this about.'

From what I had read, this communist guerrilla group now seemed to make things happen through intimidation, threats, abductions, beatings, torture and summary executions – all in the course of a so-called popular 'people's war'. They had indeed, as Abhay indicated, emerged from a 1967 peasant uprising against the forcible seizure of land and confiscation of food grains (in the West Bengal village of Naxalbari – which gave them their name). Over the years, many of central India's tribal people in Gadchiroli have become Naxal guerrillas – a response to their marginalisation by a government that has denied them rights to the produce of their traditional lands and threatened both their livelihoods and their way of life with dams, irrigation projects, mining or forest clearance.

Nearly fifty years later, in the current 'revolution', their influence is largely felt through careful selection of their victims: village leaders and other persons of high standing, and those who either refuse to cooperate with them or are suspected of being police informers. The Naxals chase the police and the police chase the Naxals – and both are brutal. In the ongoing cycle of despair and violence, the ordinary lives of civilians are too often collateral damage.

'Today they definitely cause enormous stress to people,' Abhay continued. 'Locals used to say we live under two governments. During the daytime, it is the Bombay *sarkar* (state government); and during night-time, it is the jungle *sarkar* – which means Naxalites. They do not move during the daytime very openly. At night-time they come to a village and ask for money, food, shelter, these young boys or girls.'

Revenge killings are intentionally demonstrative, brutal, public acts of terrorism. 'Sometimes they ask even family members to witness it,' Abhay said. 'Because of the Naxalites and the fear they cause, it is difficult to get our people to go to tribal villages. It's risky also, but we do not have any security. No security will work against them. Plus it is not our philosophy to use arms. But we really have two kinds of security. One is that being part of the medical profession itself offers some protection. And secondly, when Naxalites say to villagers things like, "We should stop these SEARCH people, they might be American agents," then the villagers tell them, "But then who will provide us with medical care? We want them to stay." And usually they are not really pressed after this. We get a little trouble sometimes, but nothing serious.'

Rani and Abhay might be impressively relaxed about the presence of the Naxalites and ongoing police battles between the two, but there are other aspects of life in Gadchiroli that they find much more serious. When they came here – in fact, the very reason they came here – there was a gaping lack of healthcare. Its rural people, and particularly its tribal women, had been living completely under the radar of India's medical system.

'In India the doctor to patient ratio is one doctor to two thousand population,' Abhay told me. 'The World Health Organisation norm is one doctor to one thousand population. So I wouldn't say we are *very* bad, but there is an enormous concentration of doctors in our cities and in the private sector. I don't know the number off-hand but in India, in rural areas, the ratio is nearer one doctor per ten thousand people. So there's a lack of manpower, there's a lack of supplies and medicines; the governance is poor. Usually when I discuss with the politicians they say there is no point putting in more money because our system cannot convert it into effective services.'

Talking to Abhay gave me a fascinating insight into rural medicine in India. In a place where good medical care was almost entirely absent, the power of access to doctors was incontestable. In a sense, medicine triumphed where firearms had failed – SEARCH was off limits to terrorist attack because, for the rural people and tribals alike, it was the best healthcare offering in town. But Abhay's description of the political inertia was disheartening. It reminded me of what had motivated Devi Shetty to set up Narayana Healthcare. There had been criticisms levelled at Shetty for working outside the system, but from what Abhay was saying, the system was broken. On average, countries spend around six per cent of gross domestic product (GDP) on health provision. In India's 2014–15 budget, the percentage of its GDP invested in healthcare actually dropped, from 1.2 per cent to one per cent, despite already being one of the lowest in the world (the average spend in developing countries is 2.8 per cent).

Doctors and politicians alike seemed to be raising the same concerns – even if they increased the amount of spend, would it really deliver medicines and care to the people it was intended for? The government's solution is still far from evident but, like Shetty, the Bangs' solution was to do something themselves by identifying an area of greatest need and then trying to address it.

Building links and gaining trust in the Gadchiroli jungle, however, would not be a simple matter of superimposing an urban medical perspective on their rural patients. As outsiders, especially when working with tribal people, trust would play a key role in the relationships between SEARCH staff and the locals. Fostering such trust would require a deep understanding of what rural life was like, the problems that really afflicted the communities, and getting to grips with superstitions and existing ideas about health and disease. And because there was no hospital in the place the Bangs decided to work, healthcare would have to start in the community, not in the clinic.

As Rani told me, even as students both she and her husband had been keen to specialise in community medicine. At the start of their careers, when they worked in another, better served part of Maharashtra (Wardha, around 200 kilometres away), they realised their training had prepared them only for a clinical setting. But they found that conditions in a hospital and conditions in the community were very different. As Rani said, 'In a clinic, as a doctor, I am in a powerful position. Patients come to me. When I talk to the patients, they have to listen to me whatever I say. But when I talk about community health problems, then the people have the upper hand.'

Improving the health of communities is a complex business – probably particularly so in close-knit communities, where social structures and tribal or family bonds are incredibly important. In the Gadchiroli communities, long excluded from adequate external healthcare provision, people had their own approaches to maintaining health and ameliorating disease; and health advice was passed through faith healers, mothers-in-law and other family or wider group members. The diseases people were contracting and dying from were not well documented by such communities, so the Bangs decided to make their own enquiries. First, though, they had to learn some appropriate epidemiological techniques and research methodologies. In doing so, they noticed that almost all the research into India's health problems had been done by non-Indians. 'So we thought, why can't we do the research?' said Rani. 'Here we were already close to our community.'

As she spoke, villagers from the remote jungles of the Gadchiroli district were filing into the jungle camp's consulting rooms, which had been built using money given by her father and from charitable donations. For the local people, the hospital she and Abhay had set up and run, the mobile health buses and the village health workers they trained had brought unprecedented access to high-quality healthcare, particularly for the women in the area.

It was one of their early, female-focused studies, which had been done in this hospital camp, that I had partly come to see Rani about. A few months previously I had attended a global health conference in London, and been shocked by the images and statistics that were presented on maternal mortality in India. In this country where goddesses were revered, it seemed its mortal women were being sidelined in a way that had raised a red flag among health organisations, governments and NGOs worldwide. The camp's study focused on the health of mothers and newborns, and it involved the recruiting and meticulous training of nurses, midwives and community health workers, to dramatic effect.

Rani described to me how in tribal areas maternal health was worse than in other parts of India, something that had inspired her to conduct a study whose major focus was on women's and children's health. She said that, until that point, women's health was looked at only within the context of their role as mothers. This included care during pregnancy, delivery and post-partum, and family planning but excluded sexual health education, easily accessible and safe abortion services and treatment for reproductive tract infections (RTIs) and sexually transmitted diseases (STDs). Rani wanted gynaecology and sexual care to be a part of basic healthcare for these women. 'So we started with a study on women's reproductive health,' she told me.

Ninety-three per cent of Gadchiroli's million inhabitants live outside the area's urban settlements, and more than thirty per cent of them belong to the Gond tribe. The Gonds are technically divided into three types – the Maadiya Gond, who live in the hills, and are said to be the least changed by the trappings of modern life; the plain-dwelling Gonds; and the Raj Gond, so called because they are said to be the descendants of the old kings of the tribal area. Such old divisions seem to have blended latterly, and though many now dress and live in ways that are indistinguishable from the general Gadchiroli population, tribal villages still run under Gond traditions. There, food is mainly hunted or gathered and, unlike the more modest, full-length dress of other rural Indian women, many Gond ladies wear their saris short and without blouses, and their bodies are decorated with tattoos.

While no one in rural Gadchiroli would be considered well off by urban, middle-class standards, rural villages in which Gadchiroli's majority (non-tribal) population live have concrete or brick-built houses, a few vehicles, schools and other infrastructure recognisable from any small town in India. The tribal villages are striking by contrast. They emerge like mirages from the forest, in a clearing but never far from the trees, because the jungle provides tribals with food, bamboo and other essentials. The village itself consists of twenty or fewer thatched, one-storey mud-brick houses, open communal spaces and a few shared, free-running livestock.

There is no money to speak of here – certainly no disposable income. Food and services are shared within and among villages. Tiny incomes are generated from forest resources, more so since a recent Government of India Forest Department decision to allow tribals to benefit from the natural produce of their traditional lands. But these villages are *very* remote, which means that as well as being poorer than their non-tribal neighbours, tribal women are often less well nourished (an effect exacerbated by restrictions on what pregnant Gond women are allowed to eat) and very, very far from hospitals should an emergency arise.

Rani's early studies found that nearly fifty per cent of the women they studied had an RTI. Interestingly, these RTIs were due not just to AIDS or sexually transmitted diseases, but also to poor nutrition. General malnutrition, and conditions such as intestinal parasites and dysentery that prevented the villagers absorbing nutrients from what they did eat were rife, as was the lack of dietary vitamins important to reproductive health. Diet-related and genetically transmitted anaemia was rampant, and there were also other infections introduced during homespun surgery or giving birth in septic conditions. Even though abortions had been legal in India since 1972, unlicensed abortions persisted owing to a dearth of appropriately qualified medical staff, resulting in some truly horrific infections.

There were also mental health issues and domestic abuse. Women often saw alcoholism among their men as the most troubling of their problems. Drunken husbands brought home STDs and the beatings they gave their wives sometimes ended in a miscarriage. Rani soon realised there was much more to women's reproductive health than pregnancy and childbirth. The data she gathered made a significant policy impact across the globe, so much so that now a similar emphasis on reproductive health has been accepted all over the world.

In order to provide the kind of wide-reaching care that would be able to treat and document as many reproductive health problems as possible and, importantly, generate an environment of trust in which rural and tribal women would feel at ease to discuss these issues, SEARCH trained local men and women to be health workers. The programme has been a success: in 2005, when the Ministry of Health's National Rural Health Mission began their Accredited Social Health Activist (ASHA) programme, it quickly took up Rani and Abhay's system of home-based care for newborns. The acronym ASHA also spells the Hindi word for 'hope', and it involved training one sufficiently literate person (nowadays generally a woman) per village in India's rural areas in basic medical skills, allowing them to provide primary, as well as some more complex, care to the community.

In the ministry-led, publicly funded scheme, there are currently 900,000 ASHAs across India. All of these women fill an unmet need, and the government officially recognises that critical to their success are replenishment of their medical supplies, their timely payment, regular support meetings, provision of transport for them and links to their nearest functional health facility. Unfortunately, the first three points seem not to be universally implemented, and pose a challenge for these women to continue their services. In Gadchiroli, where the operations are managed closely by the Bangs and their colleagues and cover a much more manageable geographic area – the ASHA system, which they now call *arogya doot* (health bringer) is an effective and efficient one. More than thirty intakes of these workers have now graduated from the Gadchiroli training programme.

One of the first interventions they implemented was home-based newborn care. At that time, many babies were dying from preventable deaths: young mothers in rural households either did not know how or did not have the resources to prevent them. When Rani and Abhay started, out of every thousand live births, 120 were dying before they reached the age of twelve months. They discovered that the main cause of this was pneumonia, and there was no healthcare available in rural areas for what they knew was a treatable condition. Through a combination of intervention by trained health workers and an improved immunisation programme, the infant mortality rate dropped by a third.

That was good, but for the Bangs, not good enough. 'It was not going down any more,' Abhay told me, 'so we again looked into that ... we realised that sixty per cent of the deaths were happening in the first month.' Despite the lack of specialist facilities such as neonatal care units and incubators, Rani and Abhay gradually managed to force down newborn mortality from eighty per thousand to twenty-five. He showed me one of the innovations he had introduced – an ingenious piece of equipment designed to help women with no education diagnose a lethal condition when no doctor was available. 'This is sort of an antique piece now,' he said as he explained to me how it worked. It looked very much like a child's toy, part abacus, part sand-timer, with a row of ten beads, nine blue and one red.

'So this is a one-minute sand timer, now this is for a newborn baby, and this is for an infant or toddler,' he said, pointing to one of the two rows of parallel beads along the 'abacus' part of the wooden device.

'According to the WHO guidelines, a baby up to the age of two months has got a respiratory rate which is sixty [breaths per minute] or more – for an infant or toddler, have a respiratory rate of fifty or more. Now our *dais* (traditional midwives) could count up to ten. So ...'

He turned the 'toy' upside down, and the sand started flowing downwards.

'You count the child's respiratory movement – for every time the child's chest raises, that it takes ten breaths, we move one bead. Now if before the sand has passed – which means one minute has completed, if you have had to move the [last] red bead ... it is pneumonia. I found that in eighty-two per cent of cases, the diagnosis matched. But this was twenty-seven years ago. Now we have selected one *arogya doot* in every village to become a community health worker, and she will be trained to use a wristwatch and actually count the child's respiration.'

The wristwatch was part of a health workers' kit carefully designed by Rani. Simple yet effective, it also included a thermometer, aspirator, scale, medicines, syringes, antibiotics, blankets and a warm sleeping bag.

I had learned that one of the traditional practices of tribal women was to leave babies naked for their first month. Until the baby's naming ceremony, a new mother and her baby would live in a small basic shelter, built for her outside the family home. The naming ceremony required a substantial outlay to provide food and alcohol for the entire village, consequently the mother and child could be left there for a long time. In cold weather, some of the newborns stood little chance.

In a nearby village I watched Anjana Uikey, the local tribal SEARCH health worker, as she skilfully demonstrated the procedures Rani's team had trained her in. Anjana's house was entered through a small courtyard garden filled with flowers. Petite, with jet-black hair, glasses and a pretty green sari, she offered me a chair in her main living space among a trolley of vegetables, kitchen utensils and rolled-up sleeping mats. As I sat, she rolled out a mat on the floor, piece by piece laying out the kit Rani had assembled. Anjana showed me how she used each item, wrapping a demonstration doll in a blanket; telling me how she would teach young mothers to use the sleeping bag and do the same. Her own children had been delivered at home, and since 1995 she had gone to SEARCH every three months for four days of refresher training, and to top up her supplies.

Anjana's meticulous work, and her conscientious way of thinking about what she did, were clear from our conversation. 'I enjoy my job,' she told me. 'People respect me now. When I see children playing around the village, I feel proud, because I helped them be born safely, I made sure they were not at risk of pneumonia and diseases.' And if they were at risk, Anjana also knew she had helped to avert what was now, for her and the mothers with whom she worked, preventable suffering.

In the following days I went to other tribal villages with the rural health mobile medical unit, travelling with Rishikesh Munshi, a young doctor from Nagpur. Along the way we talked about what it was like to work there, and the ailments he had commonly seen. Rishikesh's friends and family thought him crazy, leaving the city with a good medical degree to work in the terrorist-ridden jungle. 'But I didn't want to sit behind a desk,' he told me. 'I wanted to actually work closely with the people.' In his student postings in government hospitals he had seen at first hand the gross inadequacies of the infrastructure and the desperate lack of equipment, medicines and manpower. 'The doctors only turned up for two hours in the morning,' Rishikesh said. 'Instead of doing their afternoon shifts, they went to work at their private practices.' I asked him if they were being paid a full-time wage by the government. 'Yes,' he said. 'It is very unethical. But the nurses were wonderful. Everything I learned there I learned from them. Actually, I learned to do stitches from the ward boy. He was so used to there being no doctors available that he had taught himself.'

Though Rishikesh and the mobile unit were well resourced and staffed by trained and dedicated medical personnel, the patience and resourcefulness he had had to develop during his rotations must also have proved useful. He was wonderfully calm and jovial, even when our vehicle broke down on a narrow road in the thick of the jungle. As we sat on the edge of the forest in the forty-four-degree heat, he recounted more tales of conditions in rural hospitals.

When we finally reached our destination, the nurses and registration staff set out their log books and medicines under the veranda of one of the tribal village's twenty or so huts. This was a typical settlement of around 200 people, located in a clean and beautiful jungle clearing. In the distance, I could see a circular mud wall that had been raised up to demarcate it. A few goats, pigs and cows were amusing themselves; some small boys were doing the same.

'The cows are like dogs here,' Rishikesh joked. 'I've seen them jumping over fences and playing like pets. The tribals don't drink their milk because they say an animal's milk is for their babies. They only rarely eat their meat. They just keep them on the off chance that a bull might be produced for the rice paddies, I think.'

As our van played jolly film songs through its speaker to announce the medical team's arrival, the SEARCH-trained tribal community health worker set up a couple of day beds for patients to sit on. Several children and deliciously chubby babies arrived with their mothers – women with striking high-cheekboned faces and tattooed skin, wearing short saris. 'A lot of the children have ringworm and scabies,' Rishikesh said. 'Sometimes their hygiene is not good – we advise them on keeping clean as well as giving medications.'

As the nurses recorded the weight and blood pressure of each new arrival, Rishikesh carried out routine checks on newborns, examined children with various infections, elderly patients with hypertension and women with back and limb pain – the consequences of the hard labour they did in their homes and in the forests. Others had diarrhoea or pneumonia, tuberculosis, leprosy, STDs, intestinal worms, or hereditary sickle-cell anaemia – a consequence, ostensibly, of the historical prevalence of malaria in the region. The forest can be a dangerous place: people fracture bones falling from trees, mosquito bites are potentially lethal and snakes – cobras, vipers and kraits – are a constant terror once the monsoon rains begin.

But while the babies were well nourished, the women were not. 'I've seen mothers who weighed thirty-five kilos give birth to normal weight babies,' Rishikesh said, prescribing yet another fifteen-day course of vitamins and iron to yet another anaemic mother.

Rani had also told me how ideas of pregnancy and birth influence tribal women and how she has had to allow for them. 'Once,' she told me, 'I asked a group of traditional midwives about stillbirths. Everyone denied ever seeing one. At first I thought they were trying to protect their reputations, but then I realised that their concept of delivery is different from ours. To them, the baby pulls itself out rather than being pushed, so all babies must be alive when they are born, even if they then die immediately. They also see large babies like obese adults – lazy – while lean babies are considered active. So they told me not to tell a woman to take iron or calcium to increase their babies' birthweight; tell her instead that it will make her a stronger mother. It is a different way of looking at birth.'

Getting women to talk about pregnancy and what ailed them was also still a work in progress. In the village, Rishikesh and I talked more as we watched the nurses at work.

'Every worker should be trained to do everything here in case one day we don't have a member of the team,' he told me. 'The nurses and midwives know how to properly register patients and dispense medicine. We want the nurses to be able to do more too. Most doctors here are men, but we saw that reports of gynaecological problems went up twelve times after our female nurses were trained to collect medical histories.'

I couldn't stop staring at a particularly beautiful baby who had a strangely symmetrical, dotted pattern on the top of its head. Our tribal colleague from SEARCH told me it could be the remnant of some herbal hair oil, but it looked too perfectly patterned. Rishikesh and I speculated that it could be a tattoo placed there as a talisman or intervention against pain or disease. 'Once I saw a baby with thirty-seven burn marks on her stomach,' Rishikesh told me. 'The baby had had a distended abdomen, so its parents took her to a vaidu [a spiritual healer] for treatment, and he burnt her with a hot iron.'

The years of isolation and the lack of access to health services in these forest villages had lent credibility to the magic of faith healers and the rumours of witchcraft. It wasn't just the remoteness, the snake- and malaria-infested jungle or the terrorists that made access to healthcare more difficult for tribal people, or the fact that in general doctors do not want to go there. There was also a double dilemma – not only was there a lack of facilities, but Gond culture did not encourage them to seek early medical care, because they have their own spiritual healers, their belief systems and their (sometimes lethally dangerous) superstitions. Most of the vaidus to whom tribal people turn employ mantras, tantras, magic – and spiritual healing. Rani had told me that although occasionally they also use some herbs, those are secondary to the spiritual healing. That spiritual mystique was what gave them power over the minds, and bodies, of their people.

Rani's work had also unearthed some extremely distressing stories resulting from the influence of the vaidu and traditional beliefs of the tribals. Some of the rural people liken acidity in the stomach to a growling cat, leading to the logic that since cats are afraid of fire, branding the stomach with a hot iron will drive the problem away.

Until recently, it had also been traditional to bury a baby when its mother died, since there was no system of adoption and therefore no one to take responsibility for the child. Rani had also been told of the sacrifice of a six-year-old boy. His mother was a traditional midwife whom Rani had herself trained. Despite the mother's protests, the village community, including his father, slit the child's throat, soaked nails in his blood and sold them to people who put them into their paddy fields to increase their yield.

Through SEARCH, Rani had been able to prevent other

human sacrifices, such as of a man alleged to have used black magic to make a neighbour ill. But many slipped through the net. Though Gond girls have a degree of autonomy before marriage (choosing their husbands and receiving a bride-price, the opposite of the dowry system in wider India), tribal society could at times be surprisingly brutal to women, especially those who were outspoken. In one horrific case, a woman was declared a witch and held responsible for the constant illness of a relative's daughter. She was hit in the stomach with a stick and with shoes, had her clothes torn off and was forced to drink another woman's menstrual blood. Her daughter was convinced that her mother would certainly have been killed, had she not been there to plead for her.

Throughout our conversations, Rani and Abhay always emphasised that the challenges to the health of India's women were far, far broader than simply the danger of dying in childbirth – something the outside world focuses on to an almost obsessive extent. The women of Gadchiroli, for example, were at risk for multiple reasons: poor nutrition, poverty, their husbands' violence and alcoholism and the harmful interventions of spiritual healers, apart from the lack of trained medical professionals and adequate health facilities.

I had realised by this point in my travels that public hospitals in India were in the main badly resourced in terms of funding, equipment and trained staff, and that there were huge variations in quality of care depending on what state you happened to live in, and whether you lived in the city or the countryside. The Millennium Development Goals India signed up to in 1990 of bringing down child mortality by two-thirds, achieving universal access to reproductive health and, by 2015, reducing maternal mortality by seventy-five per cent have yet to be achieved.

SEARCH had found a way to commission rigorous studies in difficult environments, gather evidence, make best use of existing resources and provide robust ongoing training for local people who now served as effective and efficient health workers. They had also collaborated with NGOs in other parts of Maharashtra to replicate their Gadchiroli methods, and there, too, have helped to cut newborn deaths by fifty per cent, a success rate that other tested methods such as micro-nutrient fortifications for malnourished children have been unable to match. Their work has been commended by *The Lancet*, the WHO and Unicef, among others, so I was curious to know how far the government of India had taken the Bangs' findings on board, or what broader improvements were happening in order to achieve its goals, especially in terms of the widely reported scourge of maternal deaths in India.

'We have also studied mother's deaths,' Abhay told me. 'You might consider this heretical, but the fact is that maternal death is a very rare event.' I knew that the Millennium Development Goal target for maternal deaths was 103 for every 100,000 births. Surely India's rates were far higher than that? 'Today the maternal mortality rate in India is 178,' Abhay continued, 'which means, out of one thousand deliveries, there are under two maternal deaths. So if you ask village women, they are not much going to talk about maternal death: they are more likely to talk about difficulties or complications during labour ... It's not noticeable – for them, snake bite is more dangerous.'

Abhay's point was that, while maternal health is, of course, a major issue, looking at the numbers alone did not make sense in places like Gadchiroli, where there were far greater and more common problems than death in childbirth per se. Addressing the risk factors that can lead to such deaths would surely be a wiser strategy. 'It's looking after women before the birth, during the birth and after the birth. Monitoring is very important during pregnancy,' Abhay said.

But government policy in India continues to focus on

the birth itself – or, more specifically, where it should take place. There has recently been a drive to get women to give birth in hospitals or clinics, away from their homes and families, a reversal of a failed initiative begun in the 1980s that had promoted the use of traditional *dais* (community-based midwives).

'The *dais* received initial training,' Rani said, 'but never ever any retraining. It was only an effort on paper. Their kits were not replaced, they were not given any medicines, any equipment, nothing. And in spite of that, the *dais* were working.'

The government had promised they would be paid, but many never received a single rupee, according to Rani. The women they assisted also stopped paying for their services, since the *dais* were now supposed to be earning a state wage. 'So they had no income,' explained Rani.

I recalled how official reports of the ASHA programme cited as reasons for its success exactly the points that had been overlooked with *dais* – regular meetings, replenishing of supplies, timely payment. Because of these miscalculations or misdemeanours, the officially backed *dai* system died a death and, worse, a traditional practice that might have functioned as well as SEARCH's *arogya doots*, began to be blamed by medical communities for a high level of maternal mortality. My own research supported what Rani told me: when I had mentioned *dais* to gynaecologists in an urban Bangalore hospital a few months earlier, I had been told that they were unhygienic in their practice and untrainable.

In 2005 the government's *dai* strategy was replaced by a programme known as Janani Suraksha Yojna or JSY ('the Protection of Mothers Project'). The initiative was created under the National Rural Health Mission to reduce maternal and newborn deaths by promoting institutional delivery among poor (rural) pregnant women. Participants were offered a variable cash incentive (around Rs1,500), to help cover the cost of travel and neonatal supplies.

This was fine in theory, but there were serious practical problems, not least the fact that many rural women have no proper hospital they can go to, just a local public health centre or subcentre. 'There are often no doctors in those places,' Rani said, 'and the nurses don't always know how to manage the complications. They don't know even how to give stitches, if there is a tear during the delivery. Things are so bad.'

The second point concerned the cash incentives. In 2014 eleven young women in rural Chhattisgarh died after taking part in a mass sterilisation campaign they had been paid Rs1,400 (£14) by the government to participate in. A careless attitude by staff towards incentivised patients was blamed, and the point was also made that, when women who are living in poverty are offered money to undergo a procedure, they are likely to accept whether they want to or not. Photographic evidence of the sterilisation victims made it hard to disagree. These were very poor women who might easily have made other contraceptive choices. As mothers lay dying, their children sat helplessly next to them on the hospital beds, while other relatives sat close by on the floors of those sparsely equipped wards.

Sadly, this was no isolated incident. Over the years, thousands of women have died following unnecessary admission to ill-equipped institutions with under-trained or negligent staff. The issue was further complicated by corruption. Rani described to me how many women who took up JSY's offer either received no money, or, on the other hand, spent it on things for which it wasn't intended. Payment was made only to those holding a BPL (Below Poverty Line) card, but, as Rani explained, 'Actually we see government employees with BPL cards and the real poor – the people who should have that money – they don't get one. And those who do get paid – that money is supposed to buy food and medicines for the mother and the child, but gets spent on household items. Furniture and other things like that. And so the total purpose is lost.'

The combination of forcing women into hospital and giving them cash incentives also seemed to be having another unwanted side effect: a rise in unnecessary caesarean operations. Abhay thought this could be due to the more intensive monitoring of hospitalised women during labour. 'There may be several false alarms, and doctors get panicked.'

He also believed that some women were undergoing procedures needlessly for altogether more sinister reasons. Some obstetricians or doctors, aware that their patient will soon be in receipt of a JSY payment, will tell the family that their relative requires an entirely unnecessary caesarean. 'They say, "This woman is in danger, and an emergency operation must be done. If you pay me three thousand rupees, I can help you." Of course, every woman in labour looks to the family like she's seriously ill, so they pay up, even though state hospitals are supposed to provide free care. Some of our own workers have been victims, even though SEARCH is quite a well-known organisation – such payment is still so common that they don't care.'

I wondered whether Abhay had been overstating the problem but, as I was later shocked to discover, what he had told me was no isolated series of incidents.

More than 800 million Indians have little or no access to modern healthcare, and statistics for 2013 show that there were seventy-two suicides daily by those with illness for which they could not afford to seek help. Some part of the blame must fall at the door of the corruption rife in many state-run hospitals. Sinking into a deep depression over the basic human right of access to healthcare begins to make sense once you realise what an ordinary person – even a pregnant woman – must face. There are innumerable news stories about the desperate facilities and underhand dealings women in labour often navigate: disturbing pictures of rooms full of women on bare metal beds, the ward floor strewn with blood-stained cotton and miscellaneous rubbish, loose wires dangling lethally from the walls. There were stories of payment demanded not only for caesarean sections, as Abhay had said, but also for drugs and bandages, food, gloves, blood tests, examinations – charges were even levied in order for the woman to receive stitches *after* she'd been cut, or to receive the government benefits she was owed. One couple was asked to shell out Rs500 as the going rate for having had a son delivered, and another woman was charged Rs750 (three weeks' salary) but died in labour, leaving behind three young children.

Government statistics reveal that, today, nearly eighty per cent of Indian childbirth occurs in hospitals. But, for a programme that has heavily invested public finances over the space of a decade, the pace of improvement has been decidedly leisurely. From 500 deaths per 100,000 women in 1996, to 212 in 2009, to 178 in 2015 – the trajectory of falling maternal mortality is showing a frustratingly steady rather than reassuringly steep decline. Certainly, through JSY there has been no rise in maternal deaths, but that might be due to a number of factors, buffered by the improved economic status, nutrition, education and progressive urbanisation of some rural communities.

Even if women don't end up on the receiving end of surgical extortion, there are still disadvantages to giving birth in hospital. Hospitalisation is not universally recommended even in Western healthcare systems – the model for this programme. Abhay reminded me of the UK's National Institute for Health and Care Excellence (NICE) guideline that moving women who have no other risk factors during pregnancy to a hospital for delivery puts them at an unnecessary risk of suffering various hospital-based complications – caesarean section, panic, hospital infections. It was a sound argument. In India, the low-risk BPL women JSY was supposed to protect could well be far better off at home. 'The advantage of moving to a hospital, if any,' Abhay said, '[is that] there is a facility for blood transfusion and a caesarean section. [But] the WHO says that only around ten per cent of women need an intervention. So for that ten per cent we are moving one hundred per cent of the women.'

'What about the big dangers, like obstructed labour or eclampsia, that can occur suddenly?' I asked.

Abhay agreed that, ideally, wherever a woman might deliver, she should have access to emergency obstetric care within two hours. This, though, was a concept very different from moving every woman to a hospital for delivery. A far more practical and, in all likelihood, hygienic proposal would be to allow a woman to deliver anywhere, but to ensure that emergency transport, and timely access to a hospital, are on hand.

'Wouldn't that demand a huge infrastructural change in India?' I asked. Sitting where I was, in a camp in a jungle, I wondered how such emergency access would be provided.

'No, that has already happened in India,' Abhay insisted. As a result of the country's economic boom and international investment, the India of the 1980s, even the 1990s, was a far distant memory in 2015. 'In the past fifteen years, there has been a growth in private vehicles, roads have improved,' he said, 'mobile phones have appeared. Every village has tractors or four-wheel-drive vehicles. So emergency access to hospital care has become much more feasible. But we are preventing the development of specialist emergency obstetric services because we are so busy managing this huge load of deliveries of women who don't really need hospitalisation but come because they are paid fifteen hundred rupees.'

What Abhay seemed to be saying was that, contrary to appearances, India's healthcare problems did not always stem from a lack of access or facilities per se, but from a failure to make the best use of the resources available. Certainly, anyone who has been to a government hospital in India will have noticed that they are already crowded beyond capacity. Abhay's point, as I understood it, was that removing unnecessary pressure on the infrastructure – be that health centres or the means of accessing them – could ensure that they were more intelligently funded and efficiently used. More importantly for the long term, the hope is also that smarter policies and targeted funding would help to give rural communities the well-equipped and well-staffed health centres they deserve – and put a stop to pregnant women being used as a commercial venture.

'Is the government listening to people like you?' I asked Rani. 'I mean, you have the evidence, you have the statistics ... the studies over the years ...'

'Previously I used to go to these government meetings and all that, I used to go to a lot of international meetings. And then I stopped going. Because it was so frustrating,' she replied. 'So frustrating. The same faces would come to these international meetings, the same women, the same representatives all from an urban elite background. Who don't have any sense of what is happening in rural areas. And they would say the same rhetoric there. The meetings would be in five-star hotels, in big cities. And then nothing happens ... So I thought instead of spending that time maybe I can help my women if I work here. That way our home-based care was taken up across India and in Nepal, Bangladesh, Pakistan and several African countries, including Malawi, Zambia and Ethiopia. Our reproductive health programme was accepted by governments all around the world. The government of India was the last one to accept it. Even though the study was done here in India.'

Though she sounded frustrated, Rani appeared determined to make some difference to healthcare in India: 'I may not be able to change the whole world, but take one step here. I may not make a revolution, but I can do some evolution using our models, and research.'

Over a period of twenty years, SEARCH has been working to change the care-seeking behaviour of the communities it serves, building a relationship with individuals and leaders. 'There was a lot of distrust of doctors to begin with,' Abhay told me. 'Gradually it changed. Fortunately, they have a very good rapport now with our team, because we work with them in two ways – we didn't really impose our healthcare model on them and, for six months, Rani and I used to conduct village meetings in village after village, and every year we organise their collective village assembly, where we ask them what they think we should be providing them.'

'This hospital was constructed after we had a series of consultations with villagers from nearly forty tribal villages,' Rani added. 'Where we are now, we get patients from Chhattisgarh [300 kilometres away], we get patients from Bastar, this all is tribal area so it is well located.'

The tribes gave many reasons for not attending state hospitals, but all stemmed from a certain fear of a type of healthcare that was largely unknown to them. They came from small, tight-knit communities; they were afraid of the size and anonymity of conventional hospitals. Because their houses were always built close to the earth, which they referred to as their mother, they were intimidated by multi-storey buildings. They were frightened by the white coats and clothes that medical staff wore because it reminded them of their dead, whom they traditionally shroud in white winding sheets.

'[Our] outpatients' department looks like a home – if you go to any tribal village there is a concept where two or three brothers build together around a veranda. We did that, and have placed an educational counter there – to explain about nutrition, about the medicines, and how to take the doses,' Rani explained.

'And they said that in most hospitals the conditions are such that it's "patients *andhar*, *rishtedar bahar*". That means that the patient is put inside the ward and the relatives have visiting times. "And we feel very insecure," they say. "The doctors and nurses come only once or twice a day, so we feel lost in the hospital." Someone even said that in this hospital, "because you have plenty of space, give us space – we'll bring our own material and we will construct our own huts". And so we built the cottages for them here. We also have a pharmacy with cheap medicine ... about a third of what they would pay elsewhere. Otherwise the prices are very prohibitive for poor patients.'

Rani also told me a rather lovely story, of one of the tribal assembly members, an educated man who suggested that the camp should host a 'wisdom bank'. He told her that as their scientists had computers, when the tribals came they would benefit from being exposed to the modern technology. In exchange, he asked Rani to deposit all their knowledge and traditional wisdom into her computers. Rani did that – for example, she told me of the deep knowledge tribal women have about trees. Almost like personal relationships, they addressed different trees as though they were family members; they knew their practical and medicinal uses. Rani collected these and other stories. As the tribal elder had said, there was a lot of traditional wisdom and knowledge. But because there was no traditional process of recording it, all of it could die with them if it were not documented.

The tribals also named the hospital – they told Rani that the hospital should be named Maa Danteshwari Davakhana (literally, Medicine House of the Tooth-Goddess, who was an incarnation of the goddess Parvati, wife of Shiva). Maa Danteshwari is the supreme mother goddess of the Gond community that the camp served, and a temple was placed at its entrance. When Rani dug deeper into why the tribal people wanted the temple to be placed there, they replied that in modern hospitals, doctors think they are the gods. But faith in their goddess had an equal importance to them in their healing. 'The inauguration of the hospital was done by the main priest of the group of sixty or seventy villages,' Rani told me. 'In that inaugural speech the tribal leader said that this hospital does not belong to the prime minister; it doesn't belong to the president of India, this doesn't belong to Rani Bang, it is our hospital. And every year we have that tribal assembly still.'

Before I left, I walked around the expansive forests in which the hospital, uniquely modelled as a tribal village, was built, and I spoke to some of the patients who sat outside their huts, or around the communal veranda. They looked completely at home. As I sat next to a woman under a tree, she began telling me how much she liked this hospital compared to the government-run institute in Gadchiroli town. 'This one is further for me,' she said. 'But I prefer it here a lot. Before, I used to go to our local doctors if I had an infection or a fever. They used to give me tablets and one or two injections, but they never worked, so I came here. At the government hospital they will treat us, but we don't get well. I like the doctors and nurses here. And I don't know why, but here, the treatments work.'

8

Rewiring the Brain

'WE ARE STILL VERY FAR from mimicking the capabilities of the human brain. Our brain can learn entirely on its own, it can recognise objects in the world. I'm seeing you now the way you are now, but I can still recognise you if you were in a different light or your face was turned at a different angle. In order to really recognise your face, a computer would depend on the same image, the same angles, the same lighting. We don't know how the brain achieves this. And we are nowhere near an answer.'

From his office at the Massachusetts Institute of Technology, via Skype, Professor Pawan Sinha patiently gave me a crash course in artificial intelligence. I'd found him through an article in *Wired* magazine which gave examples of how computers can get things wrong that most humans would find simply incredible. In an airport in Manchester, for example, electronic immigration gates opened for a couple who'd mistakenly swapped passports. I thought about the strictness of passport photo regulations: no smiling, no glasses, a plain, light-coloured background, the stipulations for how to frame your face in the photo. None of this, it turns out, is for the benefit of immigration officers. Instead, it's for cameras linked to advanced computing technology, to give them their best chance of achieving something even a baby would be able to do instinctively. Like most in India and the world these days, I am rarely detached from my smartphone, laptop or tablet, happily using all the apps I can get my hands on and yet grossly ignorant of the nature of engagement with our favourite technologies. I'd rarely spared a thought for how dumb our smart tech might be, compared to the three pounds of fatty tissue we carry around in our heads.

Talking to Pawan, who had trained as a computer scientist in India before studying neuroscience in the States, it wasn't hard to see why he'd been IIT Delhi's top graduate in his year and recipient of Barak Obama's Presidential Early Career Award for Scientists and Engineers – the highest scientific honour bestowed by the White House. During our conversation, I felt as though my IQ was progressively elevating – if that sort of thing were possible – while at the same time surprised by his disarming humility. Despite being the creator of a medical and neuroscience project in India that has already offered an answer to a 300-year-old riddle about human intelligence – how our brains integrate information from our senses – Pawan made the time to talk to me at length, patiently explaining what he was discovering through this pioneering work.

One day in 2002, Pawan told me, while on a visit to his father, he left the family home in west Delhi for the day. By the front door was a pot of coins – money his mother always kept there for when she was going out, to give to those who needed it. Pawan's mother had passed away, but when he saw that his father had kept the pot, he scooped some money up on his way out. It was winter, when the Delhi air thickens with freezing fog and the temperature can struggle to get above ten degrees centigrade. From his car, Pawan noticed a woman begging. When she came over to him he saw two small children with her, around six or seven years old. 'They were barefoot, dressed in rags,' he told me. 'And it was *bitterly* cold.' As he gave them the money, he noticed the children's eyes. Both had cataracts, a clouding over of the lenses which causes blindness.

'I had always associated cataracts with old age,' Pawan said. 'I was so shocked that I tried to learn as much as I could about this. I began looking into the statistics of childhood blindness.' The numbers, like the woman's two blind children, also came as a shock: around one in every hundred Indians is blind, which adds up to between fifteen and seventeen million people. There are varying estimates of what proportion of these are children, with the largest assessment standing at 700,000. These are – though terribly sad – relatively small numbers in the context of India's total population, though the size of the figure is probably because half of all children born blind in India die before their fifth birthday. For the survivors, the cycle of poverty was almost guaranteed. 'Less than ten per cent of them will get an education,' Pawan said. 'And less than one per cent of them will be employed when they reach adulthood.'

It is particularly disturbing to learn that nearly half of these children had blindness that was treatable or preventable. For example, before 2009, India had no MMR (measles, mumps, rubella) vaccination programme, a basic childhood precaution found even in many sub-Saharan countries. When unvaccinated mothers contracted rubella, their babies were at risk of congenital rubella syndrome, which increased the likelihood they would be born blind. In young children, poor nutrition and diets deficient in vitamin A resulted in scarring of the cornea – the transparent dome-shaped 'window' that covers the front part of our eyes like a glass case on a watch and without which we would be unable to focus properly. Add to that the effects of environmental pollutants like lead and nickel in the water supply, premature birth, congenital cataracts, eye infections and the fact that all of these conditions will quite likely be missed because India has only one ophthalmologist for every 100,000 people. And that's just in the country's cities: seventy per cent of those who are blind, Pawan told me, live in rural villages. Easy access to healthcare is why we don't see children with cataracts in the USA and Europe: not because it doesn't happen – just short of three children in 10,000 are born blind in these nations, compared to just over eight in 10,000 in India – but because it's picked up and corrected in early infancy, something that was not happening on the subcontinent. The World Health Organisation's statistics say that approximately ninety per cent of visually impaired people live in developing countries.

'I returned to India after that,' Pawan continued, 'and visited a few places, in Uttar Pradesh, near Calcutta, in rural areas. I got to see how truly terrible the situation was. I was thinking of starting a personal initiative, but I realised I couldn't really help that many children on an academic's salary. Then I thought that, if I could tie it to the study of visual learning I was undertaking here [Pawan was at that time investigating how the brain recognises objects, scenes and sequences], I could tap into far greater resources. MIT was remarkably supportive. They saw the merit in this global impact.' Pawan also got the United States Department of Health and Human Services' National Institutes of Health on board to help with research staff salary costs. In addition, he secured funding from several charitable foundations and individuals in the USA and in Delhi, money which went towards paying all costs for the screening, treatment and surgery of any child who needed it. It was the start of Sinha's Project Prakash.

Project Prakash – named after the Sanskrit word for light – started its work in the rural population centres of India, within some of the most densely populated states, Delhi's close neighbour Uttar Pradesh in particular. Uttar Pradesh is huge. If it were an independent country, it would be the world's fifth most populous, with around the same number of residents as Brazil. Pawan's aim was to bring vision to blind children and, in doing so, to illuminate some of the deep questions of science. In particular, the project explores one of the greatest mysteries in cognitive science:

how our brains are able to recognise people, places and objects fast and accurately and why we have largely spectacularly failed to get machines to do the same.

'My background is computer science,' Pawan told me. 'I moved somewhat later into neuroscience. But that computing background is what propelled me to think about the mechanisms at work in our brains. How does the brain make sense of the visual world after these children gain sight? There's no explicit instruction to tell them, "That's a face; that's a chair; that's a glass." So how is the brain able to organise the world into distinct objects? That's an important question – how do we organise our sensory inputs – what are some of the important cues for the brain to do so?'

I was fascinated by the way Pawan had set up a project that provided universal benefits for everyone involved: children with visual impairment got treatment and the scientists got detailed studies of the human brain in the process of learning to see, which in turn could have enormous benefits for the study of artificial intelligence. The information gleaned from the project carried benefits previously unavailable to researchers: before, studies had largely employed non-human subjects (predominantly kittens). Studies of how vision develops can also be done with young babies, as their brains and eyes get used to the visual world, but there are drawbacks: babies, of course, cannot understand a researcher's questions and respond, but they also find it hard simply to stay awake. Project Prakash was doing the same experiments, but with older children and young adults, who were able to discuss their own impressions and experiences clearly and in detail.

Despite this, there were many unknowns when Project Prakash started out: how to find children in rural India who needed eye surgery, how to provide them with the correct care when they were found and then, given the scale of the need and the size of the country, how to provide them with the best follow-up care. Even if they managed to solve these problems, there was no guarantee that correcting the sight of the children would provide the data they needed: these children were no longer infants and nobody knew for certain whether at age seven (or fourteen, or eighteen) a child would be able to recover sight, even if the apparatus in their eyes were to be made functional. Would the brain be able to process the information coming in from newly functioning eyes, or would years of darkness have put a stop to that?

Pawan wondered about this at length. Even though his proposal was well intentioned, he had to ask whether, for children like the two he had seen hanging on to their mother's ragged sari that foggy winter day, medical help would be coming too late. After all, that was exactly what previous studies in animals all suggested: the 1981 Nobel Prize was even awarded to two researchers, David Hunter Hubel and Torsten Nils Wiesel, who had described the dramatic negative consequences on brain development of kittens when they were deprived of vision. I asked him why he persisted anyway, where others would not have bothered.

'Good question,' he said. 'As I was looking at the data on the critical periods in early life that required intensive use of the eyes and visual brain circuits, I realised there were lots of caveats you had to keep in mind. Most of the animal studies looked at blindness in one eye, whereas these children had grown up with visual deprivation in both. Although it's surprising, we know that depriving vision in one eye has worse consequences for that eye than if both eyes had been deprived together. Whether sight could be acquired after treatment late in childhood was still largely an open question … but there was enough ground still to explore.'

We spoke for some time about the education of blind people, their health and prospects, his experiences so far and what the future might look like. Our chat ended only when he had to take a call from the Dalai Lama's office.

In mid-July I travelled to Delhi to see Project Prakash for myself, twelve years after it officially began. In 2003 Pawan had approached the city's Dr Shroff's Charity Eye Hospital in Daryaganj, having heard about its outstanding paediatric facilities and that their doctors would welcome the opportunity to engage in research to learn more about how children's vision develops after eye surgery. The hospital also already had rural outreach programmes. One of the doctors I was going to see was their paediatric unit lead, Dr Suma Ganesh, who had since helped supervise Project Prakash's screening of 42,000 children in Delhi and the rural parts of the states surrounding India's capital city.

Driving in from the wide and leafy roads of south Delhi, en route to the hospital, the short commute to the old city revealed the unmistakable traces of the mighty empires who have ruled India. It is one of the reasons I have always loved this city – a twenty-minute drive in Delhi is also a journey through centuries. Its multiplicity of planned settlements have been dictated by its geography and its politics, sitting as it does between the end ridge of the Aravalli mountain range and the sacred Yamuna River; a place that Afghans, Sikhs, Persians, Marathas and Mughals claimed as their own before the British made it their capital and independent India kept it that way. Still visible in gardens, golf courses and on the sides of main roads are monumental domes and pillars and robust rubble walls, the visible commemorations of the spoils of wars and the will of gods; memorials of love, life and death and the power of commerce, apparent in the souk-like markets and shiny shopping malls.

South of what had once been Shahjahanabad, the Mughal capital, was Raisina Hill, a symmetrical new power centre commissioned in 1911 by the British Raj, with their Viceroy's Palace (now the Presidential Palace) taking pride of place on the Aravalli foothills. There were several advantages to this place, not least the fact that the views from that height were liberally studded with monuments of empires past and the tombs of Mughal emperors, the symbolism of which would not have been lost on the British. The geometric system of roads that took me from the new city into the old were created by Sir Edwin Lutyens, one of the architects of New Delhi, whose first blueprints for a Manhattanesque grid-plan were vetoed on the grounds of impracticality, for they had failed to consider the city's eccentricities – dust storms principally, but presumably also the intense summer heat that rises above forty degrees centigrade. Instead, he was encouraged to take inspiration from the grand plans of Rome, Paris and Washington DC – long avenues, classical forms. The Anglo-Indian Rome of his subsequent drafts comprised triangles and hexagons revolving around roundabouts whose spokes were richly verdant, wide, tree-lined streets, designed to accommodate, unimaginably at that time, the burden of a full 6,000 vehicles. Just over a hundred years later, I sat for a while in a traffic jam with some of the city's now nearly nine million registered private and commercial vehicles that at some point jostle for right of way on those same, shaded avenues.

Once we escaped the gridlock it was only a few minutes before we saw the red stone and rubble-built old Delhi Gate, once one of the entrances to Shahjahanabad but long since separated from the mostly destroyed city walls. Beyond it were the labyrinthine streets of the city, based on a 400-year-old layout. Inside was one of the main conduits from New to the old Delhi: the Daryaganj neighbourhood, credited for the invention of butter chicken and famous for its kitab bazaar, a Sunday market for the printed word stretching two kilometres along its pavements. It was also the home of Project Prakash, which was now based within a wing of Dr Shroff's Charity Eye Hospital, established in the old city when the government donated land and funding for its expansion from a small clinic in Chandini Chowk in 1914, only three years after New Delhi's foundation stone was laid by King George V.

The wing housing the project was completed in 1926. Its striking pink-and-red colonial-era architecture, marked prominently with the date it was built, dominates Kedarnath Lane, a road bordered by the old city's main artery on one side and the park in which Mahatma Gandhi was cremated on the other. Set back from the street within gardens, its two storeys are beautifully fronted with arcaded verandas running the length of both floors. The hospital has always been a charitable foundation and, after some turbulence in recent decades, it runs on a sustainable model in which more than fifty per cent of its work is offered completely free, supported by funding from Eicher, a major Indian commercial vehicle company (and owner of Royal Enfield, makers of the iconic motorcycles). As a result, it was recently upgraded and modernised, so that its old stuccoed wings surrounding a garden courtyard now house the high-spec technology of twenty-first-century ophthalmology.

In an office overlooking the hospital's front lawn and Kedarnath Lane beyond it, Dr Suma Ganesh filled me in on the hospital's history and how she came to meet Pawan Sinha. Dr Suma had been north India's first paediatric eye surgeon, trained by an expert who had come to India from South Africa. Until 2001, she told me, there was no paediatric ophthalmology in India, save for some scattered work in Madras and Hyderabad. I made her repeat that to me: 2001 – the year I was pregnant with my daughter – seemed barely a heartbeat ago and I found myself wondering what I would have done had we been in India at the time and she had been born with a serious eye defect. In 2001, according to the Census of India report, there were between 280,000 and 320,000 blind children in the country.

'This was the first hospital to get funding for a paediatric unit,' Dr Suma told me. 'India is seen as being at the forefront of community-based eye care. Many projects from here have been modelled in African countries. But most of it is adult-based.'

It was true that there seemed to be a proliferation of eye camps in India. There have long been numerous, long-running, widely respected ventures. Dr Murugappa Chennaveerappa Modi, the pioneer of mass eye surgery in India, began running camps in British India, in the years before independence. Like Devi Shetty's heart surgeries, Modi's prolific work in remote Karnataka villages (of around 700 surgeries a day) drew contemporary comparisons with Henry Ford. The Shankar Netralaya (temple of the eye) was another mass venture, which started in 1978 as a hospital with a missionary spirit. It is now a super-speciality institution which performs 100 surgeries a day to people of any socio-economic background. It may be that in a country of such scale and such need, no number of medical offerings is too many. But despite the number of charitable eye camps, until 2001, what Dr Suma and her colleagues noted was a particular gap that still existed. 'It was just not organised for paediatrics,' she continued. 'And children's eyes are very different from adults'. The surgery is more complex, follow-up has to be different.'

Paradoxically, one of the knock-on effects of the lack of eye care for children was, as Dr Suma and her colleagues had experienced, a level of reluctance among parents to put their children forward for surgery. After several debacles involving local or national health programmes in India – such as the sterilisation scandals – there is sometimes an underlying suspicion in rural areas of large scale medical programmes. Parents' reluctance was often well founded, based on true tales of infants who sustained irreparable damage during well-meant attempts to correct sight surgically.

Cataract removal in a child is much more complicated than in an adult, a consideration that some surgeons still failed to take into account. The procedure involves break-ing up the hardened opaque lens, then making an incision through which to remove the tiny fragments before insert-ing a new clear lens. All of this requires general anaesthetic and intensive follow-up care. Dr Suma and her colleagues told me that in rural areas there are sometimes simply no anaesthesiologists. The crucial follow-up appointments are expensive for the patients to attend, or are ignored. In addition, as I had seen throughout India, a lack of access to quality healthcare combined with poor services and corruption, and a dearth of trained doctors, well-resourced government hospitals or health insurance, led what would amount to hundreds of millions of people to seek treatment using dubious techniques or from untrained, inexperienced or superstition-based healers.

Pawan mentioned several instances in which families had relied on folk medicines and orthodox beliefs, generally with tragic results. 'I remember visiting a crowded hostel for the blind in New Delhi and meeting the residents,' he told me. 'Many of them had remarkably bad cases of corneal opacities. Upon getting their histories, I found that a common refrain was that they had been treated for some minor eye ailment – maybe an infection – by a "medicine man" in their village, which greatly worsened their condition and led rapidly to total blindness. One of the "treatments" I heard mentioned a few times involved pouring honey or even sugar crystals into the eyes and forcing the child to keep the eyes closed. It's brutal to even imagine the child's ordeal.

'Parents are sometimes told by the priests or other village elders that their child's blindness is due to bad karma, the child's or their own, in a previous life. Seeing blindness as cosmically determined fate reduces people's motivation to seek treatment.'

Even when modern medical care is involved, Pawan told me, the quality of such care can leave a lot to be desired. One case he described to me involved the siblings of a twelve-year-old girl called Poonam, who I would later meet at the Daryaganj hospital. Her brothers, Pawan was disturbed to learn, had been operated on in a hospital in the

neighbouring state of Uttar Pradesh without general anaes-
thesia, leading, unsurprisingly, to terrible complications.

For some, operations like this resulted in permanent,
untreatable blindness. And this wasn't just a problem for
children. Only a matter of months before my trip, in late
2014, a story broke in the media about an eye camp in the
Punjab in which around twenty-four elderly people lost
their vision completely after cataract-removal surgery. Conditions at that camp, the reports said, had been unsanitary,
infection had set in and the damage was then irreversible.
Sadly, this type of story was not news to Dr Suma. She
knew well how intricate the eye is, how careful surgeons
had to be to avoid causing damage or infection, especially
in young children, and also, significantly, the consequences
of poor care and practices and reliance on superstitious
belief. They would have to address both these issues if they
were to provide high quality care to those who needed it
most.

The obstacles facing visually impaired children were so
great that the hospital was forced to be more proactive in its
approach. From 2001 onwards Dr Suma had been involved
in paediatric outreach. 'That meant going further and
further out of Delhi. There was such a need and it isn't sta-
bilising,' she said. In 2001, Dr Suma told me, only around a
hundred young patients were seen at the newly opened children's unit at Dr Shroff's. By 2006 this number had risen to
8,000 and today it is around 20,000. 'Even so, some parents
ask us to defer the surgery until the children are older. We
had to do a lot of mother education. We had twenty-five
field workers knocking on doors, screening children. Pawan
saw our work on the web and approached Dr Shroff's. I
remember meeting him in the canteen of the hospital back
in 2003 when he visited us to talk about his ideas.'

Pawan's aim was to help congenitally but curably blind
children who had remained untreated, and in the process
he would gain a powerful insight into how vision develops.

Traditionally, such studies are carried out by experimentation on animals. For example, research into amblyopia, the condition widely known as 'lazy eye', involves stitching up one eyelid of normally sighted kittens or baby monkeys. Some of these would be 'dark-reared', kept in a light-tight shell, before being killed and their brains dissected for study.

It's impossible to deny that such research has provided hugely important insights into conditions that cause blindness, but Pawan's proposal for Project Prakash had the very welcome added value of supplanting such laboratory studies with a real-world problem: once the children had recovered their sight, advanced brain-scanning technology could be used to reveal any neurological changes that occurred as they regained sight and started navigating the visual world. The children would stay, with their families, at the hospital for at least a week after surgery to ensure their full and satisfactory recovery. This would also give Pawan's scientists an opportunity study the initial period of sight restoration and development, and continue to monitor it during follow-up appointments.

The technology required by Project Prakash to do all this is provided by well-equipped private hospitals in Delhi. The most expensive piece of kit – which Dr Shroff's did not have – was a functional Magnetic Resonance Imaging, or fMRI, machine. Essentially a giant, extremely powerful magnet, the technology was developed only in the 1990s and even today is rarely found outside the wealthiest hospitals or research centres.

Such machines can easily gobble up a budget of $3 million, but the value to the researchers is priceless. Rather than cutting up the brains of kittens, Pawan and his team can use the fMRI images not only to see both real-time images of human brains (which is what a basic MRI machine costing a mere $1 million does) but also, by analysing patterns of blood flow and oxygen absorption in the visual cortex revealed by fMRI equipment, to infer how active (or inactive) were those regions of the brain related to vision. Put simply, the more active an area of the brain is, the more oxygenated blood it needs.

Data from fMRI machines are increasingly being used to explore all kinds of psychological and philosophical questions about the human brain and behaviour. A few years ago some of my colleagues at University College London used fMRI to investigate love (they showed people who were in love photos of the object of their affection, as well as other people they knew) and announced that they had identified four areas in the brain that were most active when their subjects became romantic. Scientists have also been looking at how our moral compass relates to brain activity – by asking subjects under what circumstances they'd be willing to push someone under a train, for example, or to judge someone's trustworthiness from a photograph. Whether the results of such studies are reliable (or, more worryingly, how they might be used to manipulate us if they are) remains an open question.

Pawan's use of the machine was altogether more practical. The subjects in his study ranged in age from children of around seven to men and women in their early twenties. Data from their fMRI studies could help determine how late into life the brain can still reorganise itself. In addition, Pawan and colleagues at MIT, as well as his former student Dr Tapan Gandhi (now teaching the first ever neuroscience programme at IIT Delhi), planned to look at whether other senses, like touch or hearing, had hijacked the parts of the brain usually reserved for processing vision.

As well as just picking out the 'visual' elements of a scene – shape, colour, location – the brains of sighted people connect visual perception with sound, smell, touch and taste. When I met Tapan in his office at IIT, he illustrated how effortlessly our brains cope with multi-sensory tasks. He showed me two cartoon-like images – one that looked like a cloud, the other like a spiky explosion. They reminded me of the Mr Men characters Mr Daydream and Mr Sneeze.

'If I told you that one of these shapes was called Maluma and the other was called Takete, which one would you say was which?' he asked.

I didn't hesitate: 'Maluma is the rounded cloud one,' I replied. 'Takete is the spiky version.'

Tapan told me that this is the answer that the vast majority of people give (irrespective of their native language) and asked me how I had decided. I told him Takete sounded sharp, Maluma smooth.

'The brain is very interesting,' Tapan said. 'It correlates imagery with structure. So from touch or shape we get some information, and at the same time you get other, visual information. The brain is somehow able to establish the link between haptic features – how something we touch feels – and visual features. We see how we feel the object. But the question is, how is the brain doing this job?'

For the Project Prakash team, understanding complexities like this was what the fMRI data would help them do.

Despite the amazing capabilities of fMRI machines, most hospitals have little use for the kind of detailed information it generates; data that an fMRI scan reveals over and above an ordinary MRI. It was amusing to hear one private hospital's confused response to Project Prakash's enquiry of whether they had a functional MRI machine they might borrow: 'Yes,' said the voice on the other end of the line, 'our MRI machine is functioning perfectly.'

The availability of one that was both functional and functioning was a lucky break for the project's researchers. Neither the Delhi Prakash team nor, indeed, its visiting foreign researchers had ever seen a facility quite like the one the private hospital offered. Their fMRI machine was housed in a slick room, furnished with latticed screens, low lighting and calming decorative statues of Buddha, giving it the air of a five-star hotel spa. The only drawback was that, understandably, the hospital's own patients took priority, so the machine was sometimes unavailable until the early hours of the morning. Despite this, the generosity of the loan meant that the data the neuroscientists needed could be gathered relatively easily.

Once the technology was in place, all that remained for Dr Suma and her colleagues to do was to identify those who could benefit from the treatment the Project Prakash team were offering. First, they set up ophthalmic screening camps in rural areas, staffed by a team of ophthalmologists, optometrists and healthcare workers. Those selected for possible treatment – mainly those suffering from congenital cataracts and scarred corneas – would go to Dr Shroff's for a more thorough examination, for example of the optic nerve at the back of the eye using an ophthalmoscope (little can be done to repair a damaged optic nerve) and ultrasound, and a more general assessment made to determine whether they were fit enough to undergo surgery. All being well, an operation would then be arranged.

Project member Harvendra Dhillon's job was to coordinate outreach camps and arrange transport to the hospital. He spent a lot of time travelling to villages, meeting patients and their families and at screening camps. All this took a lot of organising.

Harvendra told me of the links forged with the government of India's Sarva Shiksha Abhiyan initiative – a flagship programme launched in 2000–2001 with the aim of universalising elementary education. In 2006 there were a staggering 38.5 million children in India between the ages of seven and fourteen who were not receiving schooling. It wasn't until the Parliament of India's Right of Children to Free and Compulsory Education Act came into effect in 2010 that Sarva Shiksha Abhiyan got legal backing, with community-owned education programme rules being set out in 2011 for the state of Uttar Pradesh, in the rural areas of which much of Project Prakash's work begins. The

Sarva Shiksha Abhiyan staff helped Harvendra to publicise Project Prakash's screening dates and local community leaders would encourage attendance.

Pawan had explained to me how the screenings were not restricted by age or condition – he wanted to allow parents to feel confident about turning up with their children and aimed to give assistance – whether that might be glasses, medicines or surgery – to all who needed it.

But the criteria for acceptance onto Project Prakash's fMRI scans and scientific study are stringent. Normal vision is referred to as 20/20, which is a measure of what people whose vision is unimpaired can see from a distance of twenty feet. By comparison, poor vision, determined by the use of eye charts, is something like 20/70, meaning a person twenty feet from the chart sees what a person with unimpaired vision can discern from seventy feet.

Blindness is defined by the World Health Organisation as 20/400 vision. Prakash patients' visual function will be well below this standard. They all have had cataracts in both eyes since before they were one year of age and they all have lived with an extended period of blindness lasting eight years or more.

In Daryaganj, Shakeela Bi – Shroff's outreach coordinator and parent and patient counsellor – met me in the Project Prakash data-collection room at the hospital. For the more than 400 children and the young adults who'd come to Delhi to have their surgery done over the years and their parents, Shakeela's role had been an invaluable one. Even if they had realised that free surgery was available to them in the city, most would have been defeated by the logistics of accessing it, even though the project covered travel and accommodation costs. Shakeela made sure everything ran smoothly, also keeping in touch with the families once they returned home to organise follow-ups.

Despite her best efforts, that wasn't always possible. In one case, a boy whose mother had been raising him and four siblings singlehandedly on Delhi's streets was found to have a tumour in the eye. His mother brought him in regularly for chemotherapy sessions, until one day he simply stopped coming. Dr Suma and her colleagues eventually discovered that his mother had been arrested for some trivial offence. One can only imagine her turmoil as she sat in prison, knowing her son was without care and with no way to reach him. The child died in his mother's absence. It was a horrific story to take in.

Neither Shakeela nor Harvendra had an easy job. Both had encountered parents either reluctant to allow their children to have surgery or unwilling to attend follow-up appointments. Harvendra told me about one family in Agra, the city famous as the home of the Taj Mahal. There were five children, all with cataracts. All had been operated on at the Shroff and sent home with internal sutures in their eyes. Their parents, though, did not bring them back to get the stitches removed. 'When their eyes become red,' Harvendra told me, 'the parents just say, well, their eyes are red!'

I couldn't understand how any parent could refuse their child a chance of sight. When I asked her about it, Shakeela responded with a smile that was half pained, half ironic. What she said reminded me of the stories I had heard in the jungles of Gadchiroli. In attempting to provide healthcare to millions of people, here too it was not simply a matter of strained resources. Even where government funding exists, counter-productive handling has the very real potential to make things worse instead of better. 'There are some parents who are scared. Maybe they have heard of surgeries that have caused further damage, infection – they prefer not to have it done. Others have their kids in government blind schools. These schools are well funded, boarding, they provide everything. If their kids regain sight, they might lose this good education. Some schools don't want to lose their funding either, so need the pupils to keep attending.'

'We work with nine blind schools in Rajasthan, seven in Uttar Pradesh and three in Haryana state,' Harvendra confirmed. 'They each have between 100 to 300 students. We screen the students there to see which of them would benefit from some form of treatment. There are fourteen blind schools in Delhi. Eleven of them do not give us permission to even assess their kids.'

That morning, the Monday after Eid weekend, as the hospital became busy again after a period of uncharacteristic quiet during the festivities, Shakeela introduced me to some of the children who had come in for follow-ups or to help with Project Prakash's neuroscience studies.

As we sat together in the Project Prakash office, Junaid was the first to arrive. We chatted, first about what it was like before he had surgery eleven years ago. He waved his forearm just ahead of him – showing me that before he had been operated on he could only see lights and shadow within a radius of about thirty centimetres. Junaid had been one of Project Prakash's first patients. He was born with dense cataracts, as were his three siblings, and had spent his childhood within the four walls of his home, his parents frightened to let him out. They had made attempts to get him into schools in their home town in Uttar Pradesh, but the teachers were unwilling to accommodate him because he was blind. When he was fourteen he was identified for treatment via a screening camp, underwent cataract removal surgery at Dr Shroff's and then participated in some of Project Prakash's key early scientific studies of visual development.

Now a quiet, composed, well-educated twenty-three-year-old, he was smartly dressed and wore a stylish pair of glasses. He lived in a tiny slum dwelling with his family of six, but, despite the challenging living conditions, he had finished the equivalent of an entire primary schooling within the space of a year. We talked about how much he enjoyed learning maths and English. Studying had, of course, been a relatively recent event in his life, but he had been highly motivated to get an education at the age of nineteen, and under volunteer tutors paid for by Project Prakash his progress had been exponential.

Shakeela told me that Junaid's parents, despite fearing it may have been too late for the growing teenagers' sight to be repaired, were glad of the opportunity for his eyes to be operated on.

I asked Junaid what he thought about children whose guardians wouldn't allow surgery. 'If someone told me their children were blind because it is god's will, I would say, "No, it's a disease and it can be repaired, so why not repair it?" That's what I would tell the parents.'

It was interesting to hear that the impact of regaining sight was not something that benefitted only the children. Pawan had also written about the case of a mother of three boys, all born with cataracts. In 2012 they all received treatment. Apart from the obvious benefit to them, Pawan noted the knock-on effect on the mother, who was no longer taunted in her village as 'carrying a curse'.

Girls who are blind often fare worse than boys. Dr Suma had told me that blind girls are rarely even sent to blind schools. The ratio of enrolled boys to girls was 80/20. 'You don't even want to ask what happens to those girls,' she said, the implication being that they may be entirely neglected, or even allowed to die. At best, they were being denied an education, confined to their homes as a preferable alternative to suffering abuse outside it.

One of the fortunate exceptions had been a girl I had met at the hospital on the Eid holiday two days earlier, as she was being discharged from her follow-up. A tiny, angelic-faced twelve-year-old, almost the same age as my daughter, Poonam and her family had lived as outcasts on the fringes of a village in the Gangetic plains. Her father had a small income, despite being blind himself, with which to keep his wife and four blind children – Poonam and her three brothers. As Pawan had already told me, botched surgery in a rural hospital had made her brothers' blindness permanent, but thankfully she had not been sent there – ironically, probably because she was a girl.

A year earlier she had been screened and brought to Dr Shroff's by Project Prakash. Photos of her taken at the time show a withdrawn child, staring blankly ahead without expression, able to sense only light and shadows. But once surgery was completed, her recovery was rapid. A few days after her final operation she played a game of catch with the team. As they did for Junaid, Pawan and the team are now making plans for her to be enrolled in a good mainstream school. Poonam's ambition now she has sight is to become a doctor. 'To help other children, like you helped me,' she told the team who cared for her.

Pawan and Tapan both cautioned me that when a patient's bandage is removed from their newly cataract-free eyes there's no 'eureka' moment, no Damascene transformation, no effusive exclamation of 'I can see!' Those of us who have always had sight are able to make sense of, in Pawan's words, 'the confusing mess of colours, brightness and textures that impinge on our retinas every waking moment. We organise it into a meaningful collection of objects that transforms into a recognisable form. Because our ability to partition an image onto separate objects is so well honed that it seems effortless, we open our eyes and the world falls into place.'

According to Pawan, 'The experience of a Prakash child soon after gaining sight is different. The newly sighted exhibit profound impairments. They are unable to assemble the many regions of different colours and brightness into larger aggregations. Many features of ordinary objects – the overlapping sections of two squares or a portion of a baseball delineated by lacing on its surface – are perceived as entirely separate objects, not component parts of a larger structure. It is as if the visual scene for a newly sighted person is a collage of many unrelated areas of colour and luminance, akin to an abstract painting ... this makes it difficult to detect whole objects.'

Although this is how a newly sighted child experiences vision at first, Pawan says that their researchers then see interesting changes happening over time – in both the children's capabilities and behaviour – and in the patterns of activity the fMRI scans reveal in their brains. A recent scientific paper authored by some of the Prakash team paints a picture of a brain that remains impressively adaptable well into life. After surgery, and with the benefit of appropriate glasses, the brain seems to be able to reorganise itself quite rapidly, allowing a newly sighted child to process all the new sensory information he or she is receiving. As evidence, it's of vital importance because it contradicts earlier assertions that the brain is unable to cope with the sudden onset of visual stimulation after a critical period in early childhood. This could have a significant influence on whether blind children and teenagers are, in future, considered suitable for treatment.

Project Prakash's fMRI neuroimaging studies have revealed that gaining sight *can* modify the vision-related areas of our brains, even in people in their twenties who had been blind since birth. It has demonstrated the importance of motion, for example, in allowing our brains to categorise the world into distinct objects and from that learn to identify static faces, places and things. This is something most of us never even have to think about because we learn to see as infants. It is also something, as Pawan and Tapan have reported, that 'provides a launch pad for studies that are sure to enrich our understanding of the processes by which we acquire our diverse [sensory] abilities.' It may turn out that the scientific ramifications of Project Prakash's work could end up being no less transformative than the individual surgeries that restore sight to their subjects.

PAWAN TOLD ME that when the Delhi project started, he expected it to last five years. Just over twelve years on, he attributes its longevity to the fact that the longer the project continued, the more questions the team found to address. Why, for example, does the area of a blind person's brain that processes vision remain so flexible, despite never having been used for that purpose? And why did some children improve so much more than others, when their starting point – the blindness they had for an equivalent number of years – was the same?

The neuroscience being done in labs at MIT, Boston and IIT Delhi could also lead to 'bio-inspired design' – that is, the creation of computer vision capability that models itself on human biology. Inadvertently, the Prakash studies have also fed into other research on autism. From looking at how blind and newly sighted children navigate the world, it appears that some of the hallmark features of autism – an insistence on uniformity and ritual, anxiety created by sensory overstimulation, enhanced abilities in particular fields – may be caused by sufferers' brains not having the same predictive abilities as people without autism, the lack of which means that events can seem to happen unexpectedly and without cause. As the work proceeds, Pawan hopes it will benefit autism diagnosis and therapy.

In the meantime, as Pawan says, the most immediate and tangible impact of Project Prakash is the change it brings about in formerly blind children's lives. From a 2013 survey of ninety-three of their children, they were able to report that this improvement had had a positive impact on their independence, social integration and aspirations. But there is still a huge amount of work to be done in India if a lasting solution to the problem of childhood disabilities is to be found.

AS I PREPARED for my return to London, it struck me that the challenges and solutions to the health of this great nation are not as diaphanous as they may at first seem. Instead, they are rooted in issues that are few in number, though massive in their implications. During my travels I'd met doctors from different traditions treating patients from various cultures and religions who were suffering from a variety of conditions in environments ranging from city to jungle. Despite all this diversity, there were nagging key commonalities that rose to the surface again and again. One wonderful thread had been the seamless implementation of technology to excellent effect in a range of contexts: health innovators that are already changing lives in digital India. But solutions remained to be found in situations almost uniformly marred by an absence of a unified government programme or state regulation; insufficient or ill-considered (culturally or contextually) public health measures; a back-drop of poor nutrition and living conditions; gender-based discrimination; lack of access to education; inadequate uptake of vaccination programmes; and always a deficit of trained medical staff where they are needed most.

The task may seem inestimably daunting, but fortu-nately, as is the case for all of the forceful individuals I met during my year of travels through India's medical land-scape, Pawan is not intimidated. 'Just being a small-time good Samaritan is not enough. We cannot rely on the gov-ernment to realise something needs to be done,' he told me. 'We have to be the actors and advocates in order to make a difference. In order to make sure all children get care, we have to bring the government into the picture. The reason I am a little optimistic is I believe we will connect with the right people to get governmental resources directed towards these children. We ought to be able to attract financial wherewithal. It's a dream, no doubt. There is immense need. But here there is great goodness and the desire to do the right thing.'

Acknowledgements

THIS BOOK WOULD NOT have come into being had it not been for the curious mind of my friend George Loudon and the encouragement and interest of the Wellcome Trust's Ken Arnold and Kirty Topiwala. It has been a pleasure to work with my publishers, Andrew Franklin at Profile in London and Thomas Abraham at Hachette in Gurgaon; and my patient and brilliant editor Cecily Gayford. Throughout the wonderful journey it took to put these stories together I have also been fortunate to have had family, colleagues, and friends – old and new – to support, critique, translate, discuss and accompany me. I am incredibly indebted to you all:

My daughter, Tara Lumley-Savile for being my companion and diary secretary through the burning April heat and the sodden July monsoons, when instead of being on a Mediterranean beach like your friends you were ankle-deep in sewage in a Mumbai mega-slum. My mother, Nalini for your unquestioning support throughout, for advice with your British Library India-Office curatorial hat on; for making Bangalore home during my investigations there; and, because I was too young in 1978 to have these conversations with your father – for filling me in on the years in which he researched and taught Ayurveda in Mysore and served as advisor on indigenous systems of medicine to the government of India. I should also thank him, my grandfather, Professor Chandragiri Dwarakanath, though he is no longer with us. I am honoured to have been able to consult his prolific writings for a book of my own. My sincere thanks also to my aunt, Professor V. Sujatha at Jawaharlal Nehru University, Delhi, whose books and words and work on knowledge, health and medicine in India inspired me greatly too.

Professor David 'Flintus' Osrin and Dr 'D. I.' Nayreen Daruwalla – not quite sure how to thank you for being my guides and friends in Dharavi, I don't think Bag Foot and I ever laughed as hard as when we were eating pizza and drinking beer in the 'off-worlds' (or Colaba) with you. Your work is phenomenally creative and unforgettable and I am grateful for being allowed to be a part of that. Thank you, SNEHA staff and your impressive *sanghninis* with all my heart for sharing it with me. For contacts, advice, and useful discussions, huge gratitude to my friends and colleagues Frank Swain, Dr Sushrut Jadhav and Dr David Pencheon. Dr Guy Attewell, you will remain a hero of mine for that epic journey from Pondicherry; and Dr Nandu Kishore Kannuri, because my Hyderabad adventures would not have happened without your brilliant help and encouragement. In Hyderabad I am also grateful to my wonderfully resourceful Urdu translator, Ramal Nikhath Alwi, it was an honour to work with you and to have spent time with your family of inspirational women. You brought such magical medical worlds to life. I would not have experienced 'fish medicine' without the Wellcome Trust's Dr Shirshendu Mukherjee's wonderful tale, and it was my great good fortune to have had as my house mate Dr Lorena Fernández Montalvo, who between surgeries at the Moorfields Eye Hospital found the time to give me a much needed ophthalmology 101.

So many people I admire have given their time generously so that these stories could take shape. Thank you for allowing me into your worlds in Bangalore, Hyderabad and Maharashtra: Dr Devi Shetty, Dr Darshan Shankar, Dr Ashwini Godbole, Dr Annama Spudich, Sunoj D, the Bathini Goud family, Hakim Sultan Rasool, the Hakim Gulaam family, Anusha, Parivallal, Dr Rishikesh Munshi, Tushar Khorgade, Dr Baitulle, Dr Rani Bang, Dr Abhay Bang, Anindita Ghose, Dr Rashmi Shetty (and Upasana), Dr Satish Arolkar, and Farah Khan. From Project Prakash: Professor Pawan Sinha, Dr Suma Ganesh, Dr Tapan Gandhi, Dr Umang Mathur, Dr Paula Rubio-Fernandez, Harvendra Dhillon and Shakeela Bi, Junaid, Poonam and all the incredible Prakash children. Thank you also to all of the associates, admin staff, drivers and cooks and patients of the wonderful organisations I spent time with who made my research possible. If I have left anyone out, I apologise. You have all been wonderful teachers.

It is often painfully exposing to allow words composed in a writer's self-imposed isolation to be read and criticised, but nothing could be more important, and I would like to thank those who made time to read what was amorphous and therefore who shaped it. Somehow, when I'd barely begun my research for this book a friend and colleague at the UCL Institute of Global Health got me to read a chapter out loud to an audience of tropical medicine experts congregated near Great Ormond Street Hospital. I kept asking them if I should stop, because I knew the chapter was overly long. They insisted I read on. Thank you Dr Rodney Reynolds for getting me to do that. Not being in my comfort zone turned out to be great fun. Thank you Kate Hoyland, an accomplished author and colleague I was lucky enough to share an office with at University College London; Dr Simon Kay, my colleague and friend from our British Council days and lunch companion during our Wellcome-UCL ones, thank you for always pressing me for 'the next chapter'. Jen Franklin, for egging me on when I felt like giving up; and for wise words on the importance of non-doing. James Hampson, for his musings from Cairo which ameliorated everything (even when I was trying to catch wifi outside a tribal hut one dark, forty-eight degrees centigrade night in a cobra-, malaria-, and terrorist-filled jungle). Sorry for cutting into your guitar time by making you read my Dickensian drafts. And thank you for being my sounding board Dr João Medeiros, and for having far more faith in me than I had in myself. Your ear, eye, and that *sitzfleisch* philosophy have proven invaluable in the writing of this book. And, Jacob Singh, thank you for the debates and conversations – genetics to gyms, it was all thought-provoking, and it was fun to experience a whole different side of Delhi with you.

Though I have enjoyed it all immensely, I often wished I had more time to do a book of this sort the justice it deserves. The 'tea and petites madeleines' of my ancestry, these issues and this place, to quote Proust again, 'blended the uncapturable whirling medley of radiant hues, and I cannot distinguish its form, cannot invite it, as the one possible interpreter, to translate to me the evidence of its contemporary ...' In this work I merely present an attempt to capture at least the radiant hues – and that would not have been possible without all those I met on my travels over the last year: from my Mumbai, Delhi, Bangalore, Hyderabad and Jaipur friends (old and new), to the auto drivers and manual labourers who told me what clinics they chose and why; to the social workers, scientists and doctors reshaping Indian medicine today. Thank you all.